Pocket Mar

Osteopathic Ma

MW00988086

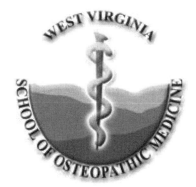

A Pocket Manual of OMT

Osteopathic Manipulative Treatment for Physicians

Editor, Co-Author
Karen M. Steele, DO, FAAO
Professor and Chairman, Osteopathic Principles and Practice
Associate Dean for Osteopathic Medical Education
West Virginia School of Osteopathic Medicine
Lewisburg, West Virginia

Editor, Co-Author
David R. Essig-Beatty, DO
Professor, Osteopathic Principles and Practice
West Virginia School of Osteopathic Medicine
Lewisburg, West Virginia

Co-Author
Zachary Comeaux, DO, FAAO
Associate Professor, Osteopathic Principles and Practice
West Virginia School of Osteopathic Medicine
Lewisburg, West Virginia

Co-Author
William W. Lemley, DO, FAAO
Professor, Osteopathic Principles and Practice
West Virginia School of Osteopathic Medicine
Lewisburg, West Virginia

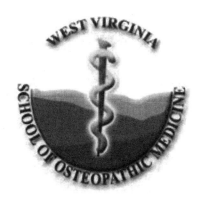

Acquisitions Editor: Nancy Anastasi Duffy
Development Editor: Kate Heinle
Production Editor: Debra Murphy
Cover Designer: Quantum Corral
Printer: Sheridan Books in Ann Arbor, MI

Copyright © 2004 by West Virginia School of Osteopathic Medicine
Copyright © 2006 by West Virginia School of Osteopathic Medicine

351 West Camden Street
Baltimore, MD 21201

530 Walnut Street
Philadelphia, PA 19106

All rights reserved. This book is protected by copyright. No part of this book may be reproduced in any form or by any means, including photocopying, or utilized by any information storage and retrieval system without written permission from the copyright owner.

The publisher is not responsible (as a matter of product liability, negligence, or otherwise) for any injury resulting from any material contained herein. This publication contains information relating to general principles of medical care that should not be construed as specific instructions for individual patients. Manufacturers' product information and package inserts should be reviewed for current information, including contraindications, dosages, and precautions.

Printed in the United States of America

Library of Congress Cataloging-in-Publication Data

Pocket manual of OMT : osteopathic manipulative treatment for physicians
/ editors, Karen M. Steele, David R. Essig-Beatty;
[co-author, David R. Essig-Beatty . . . et al.]. p. ; cm.
"Initially published in 1998 as the Mini-manual of muscle energy and
HVLA"–Pref.
Includes bibliographical references and index.
ISBN-13: 978-1-4051-0480-7 (pbk. : alk. paper)
ISBN-10: 1-4051-0480-5 (pbk. : alk. paper)
  1. Osteopathic medicine—Handbooks, manuals, etc. 2. Osteopathic
orthopedics—Handbooks, manuals, etc. 3. Primary care (Medicine)
—Handbooks, manuals, etc. I. Essig-Beatty, David R. II. Steele, Karen
M. III. Title: Mini-manual of muscle energy and HVLA techniques.
  [DNLM: 1. Manipulation, Osteopathic–methods–Handbooks. 2. Primary Health Care–
Handbooks. WB 39 P7393 2006]
RZ342.P63 2006
615.5'33—dc22

                              2005015952

The publishers have made every effort to trace the copyright holders for borrowed material. If they have inadvertently overlooked any, they will be pleased to make the necessary arrangements at the first opportunity.

To purchase additional copies of this book, call our customer service department at **(800) 638-3030** or fax orders to **(301) 824-7390**. International customers should call **(301) 714-2324.**

Visit Lippincott Williams & Wilkins on the Internet: http://www.LWW.com.
Lippincott Williams & Wilkins customer service representatives are available from 8:30 am to 6:00 pm, EST.

07 08 09
4 5 6 7 8 9 10

CONTENTS

ACKNOWLEDGMENTS

Thanks are extended to WVSOM graduate teaching assistants Derek Stone for editing and Karl Speers for adaptation of sacral graphics with permission of Kenneth E. Graham, DO. WVSOM students Aaron Kelley, Dana Quarles, and Linda Wilson contributed photography and editing. Karen Ayers of the WVSOM Department of Media Services assisted with photography. William A. Kuchera, DO, FAAO provided his unique drawings of biomechanics through a contract with Dr. Essig-Beatty for the book *Manipulation at Home: Exercises Based on Osteopathic Structural Exam* (WVSOM, Lewisburg, 2003). Gratitude is extended to Karen Snider, DO who contributed to the development of this book while a graduate teaching assistant at WVSOM through her initial concept and editing of the *Mini-Manual of Muscle Energy and HVLA Techniques* (WVSOM, Lewisburg, 2000), from which this book has evolved.

REVIEWERS

Jane E. Carreiro, DO
Associate Professor
University of New England College of Osteopathic Medicine
Department of Osteopathic Manipulative Medicine
Biddeford, Maine

John C. Glover, DO, FAAO
Chairman, Osteopathic Manipulative Medicine
Touro University – California College of Osteopathic Medicine
Vallejo, California

Kenneth E. Graham, DO
Clinical Associate Professor
Director of Hospital Care for Center for Structural Medicine
Oklahoma State University College of Osteopathic Medicine
Tulsa, Oklahoma

William A. Kuchera, DO, FAAO
Professor Emeritus
Kirksville College of Osteopathic Medicine
Kirksville, Missouri

Kenneth E. Nelson, DO, FAAO
Chicago College of Osteopathic Medicine
Midwestern University
Downers Grove, Illinois

PREFACE

The *Pocket Manual of OMT* is a concise clinical reference designed to assist physicians and medical students with applying manipulative treatment for common problems encountered in primary care practice. Initially published in 1998 as the *Mini-Manual of Muscle Energy and HVLA*, the book now includes all diagnostic and treatment skills taught in osteopathic principles and practices courses at the West Virginia School of Osteopathic Medicine, a top rated medical school for primary care and rural medicine.

This book represents a consensus statement of seven osteopathic educators developed over ten years, each of whom graduated from a different osteopathic medical school. Over the years, what we all agreed was truly important for the primary care osteopathic physician to be able to do in order to provide osteopathic manipulative care for his or her patients has stayed, and what we considered not necessary for a primary care osteopathic practitioner has been dropped.

The manual reflects the hard work and critical thinking of the Division of Osteopathic Principles and Practice at the West Virginia School of Osteopathic Medicine. For more than ten years, under the guidance of James Stookey, DO and Karen Steele, DO, this institution has focused on the two issues of teaching OP&P at the level appropriate for primary care practice, and also integrating manual practice into this setting. The manual is intended then to address these goals at a level of moderate depth as it teaches the various models. Also, a separate chapter has been added to encourage practical application of OMT in the primary care setting.

These factors should make it comprehensive, practical and readable for the clinician wanting to refresh and expand skills now that the pressures of practical exams and residency requirements are behind them. The regional organization of the material aids in researching useful treatments for specific clinical presentations and will be helpful in the clinical setting. Additionally, the manual is useful as an initial teaching tool for students since the descriptions and photos give clear, methodical descriptions of individual procedures. The standardized concise format of description allows for ready comparison of similarities and differences between models of technique applied in a single region.

This book has several unique features. It is the first manual medicine text to list indications and contraindications for every treatment, basing them on osteopathic standards of care, clinical common sense, and author experience. Two newer OMT techniques, percussion vibrator and facilitated oscillatory release, are included with descriptions and illustrations for each region of the body. Exercises derived from structural exam and OMT are provided at the end of each chapter, another first for osteopathic technique manuals.

Included in this manual are techniques labeled facilitated oscillatory release (FOR). To those unfamiliar, this represents the reintroduction of oscillation or gentle manual vibration as an activating force to complement other forces in many of the treatment models. The separate techniques are listed as suggestions or learning drills only since FOR is intended to integrate in a combined way with many direct techniques including muscle energy and myofascial release. They represent a dynamic approach to direct myofascial release and are applicable in many settings in which the treater desires to extend the range of motion beyond the restrictive barrier. A citation regarding an article in the AAO Journal is included for those who want to pursue this interest further.[1]

The *A Pocket Manual of OMT:* Use it to learn osteopathic diagnosis and treatment; keep it handy for clinical applications; copy the exercises for patients. Our goal for this book is the same as that of the first school of osteopathic medicine:

"To improve our present systems of surgery, obstetrics, and treatment of disease generally, to place the same on a more rational and scientific basis, to impact information to the medical profession . . ."[2]

We hope you will find this manual helpful to you in providing osteopathic care to your patients. We welcome your input as this manual continues to evolve.

Karen M. Steele, DO, FAAO
David R. Essig-Beatty, DO
Zachary J. Comeaux, DO, FAAO
William W. Lemley, DO, FAAO

[1] Comeaux ZJ. *Facilitated oscillatory release – a method of dynamic assessment and treatment of somatic dysfunction.* The AAO Journal 13(3):30–35. 2003.
[2] American School of Osteopathy, Revised Charter, October 30, 1894. Still National Osteopathic Museum, Kirksville, MO.

Chapter 1: INTRODUCTION TO OSTEOPATHIC DIAGNOSIS AND TREATMENT

Osteopathic manipulative treatment (OMT) is used to treat a patient problem associated with *somatic dysfunction*: Impaired or altered function of related components of the somatic (body framework) system: skeletal, arthrodial, and myofascial structures, and related vascular, lymphatic, and neural elements.[1]

Diagnosis of somatic dysfunction is derived from structural examination to identify at least one of four diagnostic criteria described by the mnemonic TART: tissue texture abnormality, asymmetry, restriction of motion, and tenderness. Somatic dysfunction is described as position of a body part, direction of free motion, or direction of restricted motion.[1] The *Pocket Manual of OMT* utilizes the latter denotation when relevant because motion restriction is more readily understood by practitioners other than osteopathic physicians.

Structural examination consists of screening to identify a region with somatic dysfunction, scanning to identify its location within the region, and local diagnosis to precisely define the somatic dysfunction. Screening tests including postural exam and gait analysis to identify regional asymmetry are presented in Chapter 2. Scanning tests and diagnosis skills are presented in subsequent chapters covering the ten regions of somatic dysfunction: lower extremity, pelvis, sacrum, lumbar, thoracic, rib, upper extremity, cervical, cranial, and abdominal/other (visceral).

Indications for OMT: OMT is defined as a form of manual treatment applied by a physician to eliminate or alleviate somatic dysfunction and related disorders.[2] OMT is indicated whenever the physician makes the diagnosis of somatic dysfunction and relates it to a patient problem. Examples of conditions amenable to OMT are listed for each technique in subsequent chapters.

Contraindications to OMT: The only absolute contraindication to all OMT is the absence of somatic dysfunction. An individual technique is contraindicated when its potential benefit is outweighed by the risk of harm to the patient. Indirect techniques in which the body is moved away from a restriction and into a position of tissue laxity incur less risk for patients with acute injuries, severe illnesses, undiagnosed problems, or fragile conditions. Direct techniques in which the body is moved into a restriction are less applicable under these circumstances. Relative contraindications are listed for each OMT technique in subsequent chapters.

OMT Techniques: Each type of manipulative treatment has principles of application which can be applied for any part of the body with practitioner knowledge of anatomy and function.

articulatory (combined indirect and direct): a low velocity/moderate-to-high amplitude technique developed by Andrew Taylor Still, MD in which a joint is carried through its full motion with the therapeutic goal of increased freedom of range of movement.[1]
1) Identification of restricted joint movement for all possible planes of motion;
2) Slow movement of the joint to its position of laxity for all planes;
3) Slow movement of the joint into its restriction for all planes;
4) 3-5 repetitions as one smooth movement until joint mobility returns;
5) Retesting motion.

counterstrain (indirect): a system of diagnosis and treatment developed by Lawrence H. Jones, DO that considers the dysfunction to be a continuing, inappropriate strain reflex, which is inhibited by applying a position of mild strain in the direction exactly opposite to that of the reflex; this is accomplished by specific directed positioning about the point of tenderness to achieve the desired therapeutic response.[1]
1) Identification and labeling tender point as 10/10 or 100%;
2) Passive positioning of the body into tissue laxity until tenderness at the tender point is reduced to 2/10 (20%) or less;
3) Holding of the position of relief while keeping a finger on the tender point location for 90 seconds;
4) Passive return of the body to neutral;
5) Retesting for tenderness and retreating with fine tuning if not improved.

muscle energy (direct): A system of diagnosis and treatment developed by Fred Mitchell Sr., DO in which the patient voluntarily moves the body as specifically directed by the physician; this directed patient action is from a precisely controlled position, against a defined resistance by the physician.[1]
1) Identification of restricted joint movement for all possible planes of motion;
2) Movement of the joint into its restriction for all planes;
3) Patient pushing away from the restriction against physician resistance for 3-5 seconds;
4) Slow movement of the joint to a new restrictive barrier;
5) 3-5 repetitions of isometric contraction and stretch;

6) Retesting motion.

myofascial release (indirect or direct): a system of diagnosis and treatment which engages continual palpatory feedback to achieve release of myofascial tissues.[1]
1) Identification of restricted tissue or joint movement for all possible planes of motion;
2) Indirect: Slow movement of the part of the body into its position of laxity for all planes and following any tissue release until completed;
3) Direct: Slow movement of the part of the body into its restrictions for all planes and application of steady force until tissue give is completed;
4) Retesting motion.

facilitated oscillatory release (direct): a manipulative technique developed by Zachary Comeaux, DO which applies manual oscillatory force to normalize neuromuscular function; intended to be combined with any treatment involving ligamentous or myofascial technique.[3]
1) Identification of tension and asymmetry related to restricted motion;
2) Initiation of stretch and oscillatory motion of the region of restriction using some tissue mass to initiate a standing (harmonic) wave;
3) Monitoring of the quality of motion response in the tissues to further localize restriction;
4) Continuation of rhythmic oscillation or modification of its force until tension is reduced or rhythmic mobility improves. Other corrective force may be combined;
5) Retesting for tension or motion.

facilitated positional release (indirect): a system of indirect myofascial release treatment developed by Stanley Schiowitz, DO. The component region of the body is placed into a neutral position, diminishing tissue and joint tension in all planes and an activating force (compression or torsion) is added.[1]
1) Identification of tension related to restricted motion;
2) Placing the joint or region in its neutral position;
3) Palpating the tension and moving the joint or region into its position of laxity for all planes;
4) Adding compression or torsion to facilitate tissue laxity;
5) Holding the position of laxity for 3–5 seconds until tension release is completed and then slow return to neutral;
6) Retesting for tension or motion.

ligamentous articular strain (indirect): a set of myofascial release techniques described by Howard Lippincott, DO and Rebecca Lippincott, DO.[1]
1) Identification of ligament or myofascial tension;
2) Pressing into or applying traction to the tense area to engage the tissues;
3) Slow movement of the part of the body into its position of laxity for all planes;
4) Maintaining the position of laxity using balanced pressure and following any tissue release until completed or the cranial rhythmic impulse is palpated;
5) Retesting for tension.

osteopathy in the cranial field: a system of diagnosis and treatment developed by William G. Sutherland, DO and applied by an osteopathic practitioner using the primary respiratory mechanism and balanced membranous tension.[1]

percussion vibrator: a manipulative technique developed by Robert Fulford, DO involving the specific application of mechanical vibratory force to treat somatic dysfunction.
1) Identification of tension or restricted movement;
2) Placing the percussion pad on an associated bony prominence with the pad oriented perpendicular to the surface;
3) Altering pad speed, pressure, and angle until vibrations are palpated as strong by a monitoring hand placed on the opposite side of the tension or restriction;
4) Maintaining contact until the force and rhythm of vibrations returns to that of normal tissue;
5) Alternate technique:
   a. Allowing the monitoring hand to be pulled toward the pad, resisting any other direction of pull;
   b. Maintaining percussion until the monitoring hand is pushed away from the pad;
6) Slow release of the monitoring hand and percussor pad and retesting for tension or restriction.

soft tissue (direct): a system of diagnosis and treatment directed toward tissues other than skeletal or arthrodial elements.[1]
1) Identification of tension or edema;
2) Application of force to the tense or edematous tissues by:
   a. Longitudinal stretch (traction);
   b. Kneading (lateral stretch);
   c. Inhibition (sustained pressure);
   d. Effleurage (stroking pressure);
   e. Petrissage (squeezing pressure).

4

3) Retesting for tension or edema.

thrust (direct): a direct technique which uses high vel
amplitude (HVLA) forces; also called mobilization wit
treatment.[1]

1) Identification of restricted joint movement for ~~possible~~
   planes of motion;
2) Moving the joint into its restriction for all planes;
3) Application of a short quick thrust through one of the
   restricted joint planes;
4) Retesting motion.

visceral: a system of diagnosis and treatment directed to the viscera
to improve physiologic function; typically the viscera are moved
toward their fascial attachments to a point of fascial balance; also
called ventral techniques.[1]

Exercise Techniques: Exercises derived from structural exam and
OMT are presented at the end of each chapter.[4] Type of exercise
prescribed depends on patient assessment, somatic dysfunction
present, and response to OMT.

position of ease: resting in a position for shortening of tense tissues
for 2-5 minutes to bring about relaxation and decreased pain; Useful
for myofascial tenderness associated with acute problems as well as
pain relief for subacute and chronic problems; Contraindicated for
acute fractures.

stretching: a steady movement into a restriction for 10-20 seconds to
reduce tension and restore motion; Useful for tension associated
with subacute and chronic problems; Contraindicated for acute
sprains or fractures, joint instability.

mobilization: a short and quick or slow and repetitive movement into
a restriction to restore joint mobility; Useful for joint restrictions
associated with subacute and chronic problems; Contraindicated for
acute sprains or fractures, joint instability, inflammation, severe
degeneration, or severe osteoporosis.

postural strengthening: a contraction of postural muscles against
gravitational resistance until fatigued and repeated every other day
to restore strength for standing and walking.

Prescribing OMT: Each treatment plan depends upon patient
preference, physician skill, history, exam findings, indications,
contraindications, and response to treatment. Exercises, orthotics,
braces, and thermal therapy can be prescribed to complement the

ss of OMT. Cold packs can be applied for 15-20 minutes
ed or painful areas to reduce swelling and pain. Hot packs
pplied for 20-30 minutes before or after treatment or exercise to
uce tension, stiffness, and ache. Pain due to hypermobility or
ligamentous laxity can be temporarily reduced with indirect methods
of manipulation but is better treated with stabilization techniques
such as bracing, strengthening, and prolotherapy. The latter, also
called sclerotherapy, uses injection of a proliferant solution into
weakened ligaments to strengthen or shorten the lax tissues. The
prescription of OMT is an art in which the physician uses structural
diagnosis and appropriate treatment to improve patient functioning
so that healing may more readily occur.

REFERENCES

1. Glossary of Osteopathic Terminology, p.1229 in Ward RC, Ed. *Foundations for Osteopathic Medicine, 2nd Edition.* Lippincott Williams & Wilkins, Philadelphia, 2003.
2. American Osteopathic Association. *AOA Yearbook and Directory.* American Osteopathic Association, Chicago, 2003.
3. Comeaux ZC. *Facilitated oscillatory release – a method of dynamic assessment and treatment of somatic dysfunction.* The AAO Journal 13(3):30-35. 2003.
4. Essig-Beatty DR. *Manipulation at Home: Exercises Based on Osteopathic Structural Exam.* WVSOM, Lewisburg, 2003.

NOTES

Diagnosis of Postural Problems

1. Dynamic postural evaluation – p.10
2. Static postural evaluation – pp.11-12
3. Scoliosis evaluation if indicated – p.13
4. Short leg evaluation if indicated – p.14
5. Correlation to regional palpation and motion testing – see region
6. Hypermobility screening – p.15

Postural Treatment

1. Heel lift therapy – p.18
2. Spinal flexibility exercises – p.19
3. Spinal mobility exercises – p.19
4. Postural strengthening exercises – pp.20-24

DYNAMIC POSTURE

1. Stand behind the barefoot patient and observe walking 5-10 steps away from and back toward you;
2. Identify areas of asymmetrical movement and decreased movement:
   a) Stride;
   b) Heel strike/toe off;
   c) Lower extremity rotation;
   d) Pelvic levelness and rotation;
   e) Trunk rotation;
   f) Shoulder levelness;
   g) Arm swing;
   h) Head levelness;
3. Common abnormalities:

   Asymmetry due to weakness;
   Asymmetry due to restriction;
   Decreased movement due to restriction;
   Neurological disorders: Foot drop, foot slapping, shuffling, wide stanced, staggering, lurching.

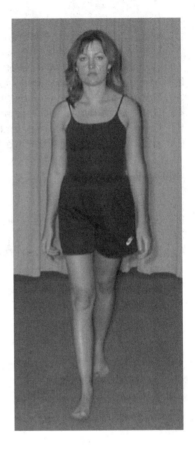

Dynamic posture

1. Stand behind the barefoot patient and observe an imaginary vertical line upward from halfway between the medial malleoli;
2. The vertical line should normally pass:
   a) halfway between the knees;
   b) along the gluteal fold;
   c) through all spinous processes;
   d) along the midline of the head;
3. Observe for horizontal levelness of:
   a) popliteal creases;
   b) greater trochanters;
   c) iliac crests;
   d) inferior angles of scapula;
   e) tops of shoulders;
   f) mastoid processes;
4. Observe for symmetry of:
   a) foot rotation;
   b) arm length;
   c) arm distance from torso;
5. Palpate:
   a) foot arches by sliding fingertips under the medial arches;
   b) Achilles tendon tension;
6. Common abnormalities:

   Foot external rotation;
   Pes planus (fallen foot arch);
   Iliac crest asymmetry;
   Pelvic side shift;
   Sacral base unleveling;
   Scoliosis;
   Shoulder height asymmetry;
   Head tilt.

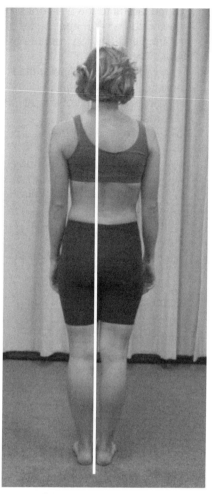

Right pelvic shift

STATIC POSTURE – LATERAL

1. Stand lateral to the barefoot patient and observe an imaginary weight bearing line upward from the anterior aspect of the lateral malleolus;
2. The weight bearing line should normally pass through:
   a) anterior aspect of lateral malleolus;
   b) middle of tibial plateau;
   c) greater trochanter;
   d) body of L3 (center of body mass);
   e) middle of humeral head;
   f) external auditory meatus;
3. Common abnormalities:

   Anterior head carriage;
   Shoulder anterior or posterior;
   Thoracic hyperkyphosis;
   Lumbar hyperlordosis;
   Anterior pelvic weight bearing.

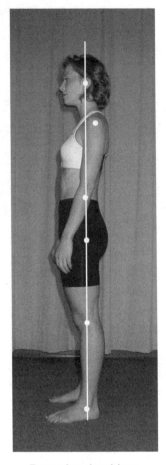

Posterior shoulders

SCOLIOSIS SCREENING (forward bending or Adam's test)

1. Stand behind the barefoot patient and ask him or her to slowly bend forward and reach for the ground with the legs straight;
2. A rib hump with forward bending indicates possible scoliosis convex to the side of the fullness;
3. If a rib hump is present, ask the patient to bend to the side of fullness;
4. A rib hump that goes away with sidebending to that side indicates a functional scoliosis while one that remains indicates a structural scoliosis.

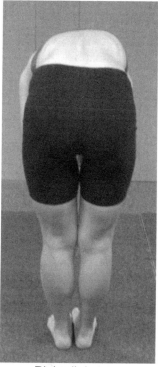 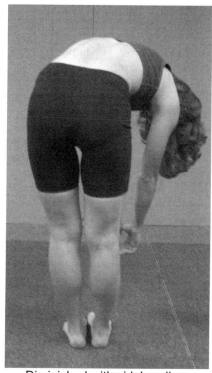

Right rib hump
(right scoliosis)

Diminished with sidebending
(functional scoliosis)

ILIAC CREST HEIGHT

1. Stand behind the barefoot patient;
2. Place your fingertips on the superior surface of the iliac crests in the mid-axillary line;
3. An inferior iliac crest indicates a relative short leg;
4. Common causes of asymmetry:

   Pes planus or cavus;
   Genu valgum or varus;
   Knee or hip restriction;
   Pelvic rotation;
   Anatomical short leg.

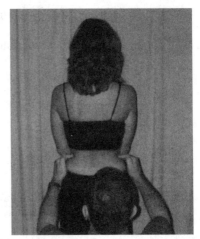

Iliac crest height

MEDIAL MALLEOLUS LEVELNESS

1. Stand at the foot of the supine patient;
2. To seat the pelvis have the patient bend the knees, lift and set down the buttocks, and straighten out the legs (see p. 73);
3. Place your thumbs on the inferior surface of the medial malleoli;
4. With your head centered directly above the ankles, compare your thumbs for superior-inferior levelness of the medial malleoli;
5. If medial malleoli are asymmetrical check ASIS levelness to determine relative leg length;
6. Common causes of asymmetry:

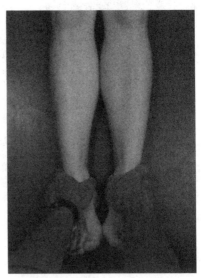

Medial malleolus levelness

   Knee, hip, or pelvis somatic dysfunction;
   Anatomical short leg.

HYPERMOBILITY SCREENING (non-dominant limb)[1]

A score of 4-5/5 indicates probable generalized hypermobility.

1. Index Finger Extension

   a) Rest the patient's palm on a flat surface and pull the index finger into extension as far as it will comfortably go;
   b) Finger extension to 90° or more = 1 point.

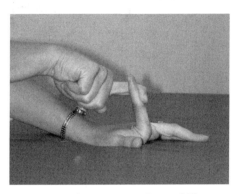

Index finger extension > 90°

2. Thumb Flexion

   a) Flex the patient's thumb toward the ventral forearm as far as it will comfortably go;
   b) Thumb contact with forearm = 1 point.

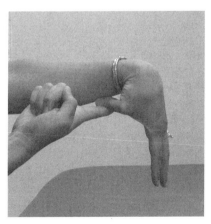

Thumb flexion to ventral forearm

3. Elbow Extension

   a) Hold the upper arm with one hand and the wrist with your other hand;
   b) Slowly extend the elbow as far as it will comfortably go;
   c) Elbow extension ≥ 10° = 1 point.

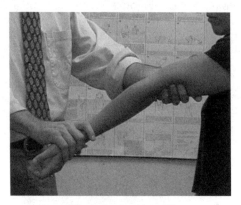

Elbow extension 5°

4. Knee Extension

   a) With the patient sitting, hold the thigh with one hand and extend the knee with your other hand as far as it will comfortably go;
   b) Extension ≥ 10° = 1 point;

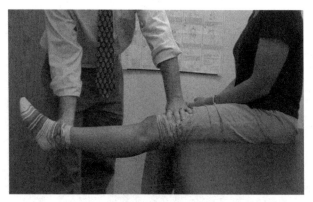

Knee extension 0°

5. Standing Flexion

    a) Ask the patient to bend forward as far as is comfortable with the legs straight;
    b) Palms flat on the floor = 1 point.

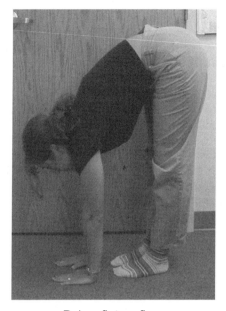

Palms flat on floor

Total Score:

    0/5 – 3/5: Generalized hypermobility unlikely
    4/5 – 5/5: Generalized hypermobility likely

HEEL LIFT THERAPY

Indications: Anatomical short leg or sacral base unleveling related to lumbar scoliosis, back pain, and other problems.

Protocol:

1. Perform OMT for lower extremity, pelvis, sacrum, lumbar, and related thoracic, rib, cervical, and cranial somatic dysfunction;
2. Insert 1/8" heel lift into the shoe on the side of the short leg except for:
    a) Fragile patients (severe pain, radiculopathy, elderly, severe arthritis, severe osteoporosis) – begin with 1/16" lift and increase by 1/16" every two weeks;
    b) Recent sudden loss of leg length (fracture, prosthesis) – begin with entire amount of needed lift;
3. Increase lift by 1/8" every two weeks as tolerated following OMT until there is iliac crest levelness with standing;
4. Up to 1/2" of heel lift can be used before foot tilt requires that any additional lift be added to the entire sole.

SPINAL FLEXIBILITY EXERCISES

Indications: Muscle tension related to postural strain, scoliosis, short leg syndrome, back pain, neck pain, headache, stress, anxiety, and other problems.

Contraindications: Acute strain, sprain, or fracture; hypermobility; undiagnosed radiculopathy; unexplained fever or weight loss.

Exercises: Do the following exercises 1-4 times a day if tolerated.

1. Hamstring stretch (p.61)
2. Lumbar extensor stretch (p.146)
3. Thoracolumbar stretch (p.147)
4. Thoracic flexor/extensor stretch (p.180)
5. Cervical extensor stretch (p.246)

SPINAL MOBILITY EXERCISES

Indications: Restricted motion related to postural strain, scoliosis, short leg syndrome, back pain, neck pain, headache, stress, anxiety, and other problems.

Contraindications: Acute strain, sprain, or fracture; hypermobility; cancer; joint inflammation; severe joint degeneration; severe osteoporosis; undiagnosed radiculopathy; unexplained fever or weight loss.

Exercises: Do the following exercises up to twice a day if tolerated.

1. Sacroiliac mobilization (p.117)
2. Lumbar mobilization (p.147)
3. Thoracolumbar mobilization (p.147)
4. Thoracic mobilization supine (p.181)
5. Cervical sidebending mobilization (p.250)

19

POSTURAL STRENGTHENING

Indications: Postural weakness related to inactivity, hypermobility, back pain, neck pain, headache, and other problems.

Contraindications: Acute strain, sprain, or fracture; unstable cardiac arrhythmia; undiagnosed radiculopathy; unexplained fever or weight loss.

Exercises: Do one of the following routines daily or every other day.

Beginner:
1. Pelvic tilt (p.21)
2. Supine lift – bent leg (p.22)
3. Prone lift – one leg (p.23)

Intermediate:
1. Supine lift – both legs (p.22)
2. Prone lift – one leg and arm (p.24)
3. Abdominal curl (p.21)

Advanced (wrist and ankle weights may be added if needed to reach fatigue by the third repetition):
1. Supine lift – both legs and arms (p.23)
2. Prone lift – both legs and arms (p.24)

PELVIC TILT

1. Lie on your back with knees bent and feet flat on the floor;
2. Roll the pelvis back by pushing the low back into the floor and lifting the coccyx (tip of tailbone) slightly upward;
3. Take a few deep breaths and hold this position for 5-20 seconds;
4. Repeat 5-10 times.

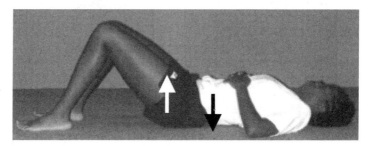

Pelvic tilt

ABDOMINAL CURL

1. Lie on your back with knees bent, feet on the floor, and arms crossed;
2. Slowly lift your head and shoulders until the head is 3-6 inches from the floor;
3. Hold your head and shoulders in this position for 20 seconds;
4. Repeat 3 times;
5. If the third lift is easy increase the time by 10 seconds.

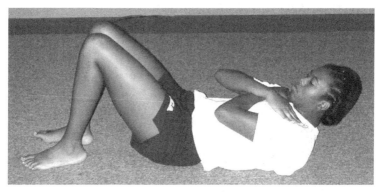

Abdominal curl

SUPINE LIFT – ONE LEG

1. Lie on your back with one knee bent and that foot on the floor;
2. Allow your bent knee to fall to the side and slowly lift the entire leg until your foot is 3-6 inches from the floor;
3. Hold your leg in this position for 10 seconds;
4. Repeat for the other leg;
5. Do this leg lift 3 times for each leg. If the third lift is easy, increase the time held by 10 seconds;
6. Do this exercise every other day.

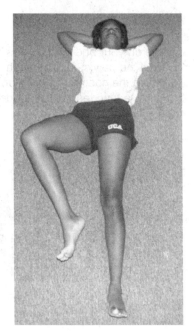

Supine lift – one leg

SUPINE LIFT – BOTH LEGS

1. Lie on your back with the legs straight and toes pointing downward;
2. Tighten your buttocks and slowly lift the legs until your feet are 3-6 inches from the floor;
3. Hold your legs in this position for 20 seconds;
4. Repeat this leg lift 3 times. If the third lift is easy, increase the time held by 10 seconds;
5. Do this exercise every other day.

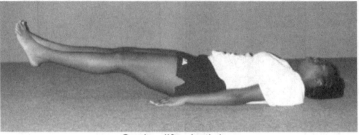

Supine lift – both legs

SUPINE LIFT – LEGS AND ARMS

1. Lie on your back with the legs straight, toes pointing downward, and arms straightened above your head;
2. Tighten your buttocks and slowly lift the legs, arms, and head until your hands and feet are 3-6 inches from the floor;
3. Hold your legs, arms, and head in this position for 30 seconds;
4. Repeat 3 times. If the third lift is easy, increase the time held by 10 seconds;
5. Do this exercise every other day.

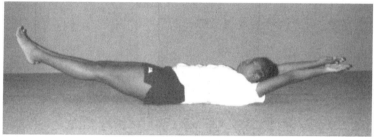

Supine lift – legs and arms

PRONE LIFT – ONE LEG

1. Lie on your stomach with the legs straight and toes pointing downward;
2. Slowly lift one leg until your foot is 3-6 inches from the floor;
3. Hold your leg in this position for 10 seconds;
4. Repeat 3 times. If the third lift is easy, increase the time held by 10 seconds;
5. Do this exercise every other day.

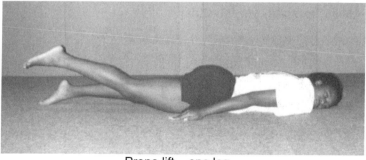

Prone lift – one leg

PRONE LIFT – ONE LEG AND ARM

1. Lie on your stomach with the legs straight, toes pointing downward, and arms straightened above your head;
2. Slowly lift one leg and the opposite arm until your foot and hand are 3-6 inches from the floor;
3. Hold your leg and arm in this position for 20 seconds;
4. Repeat 3 times. If the third lift is easy, increase the time held by 10 seconds;
5. Do this exercise every other day.

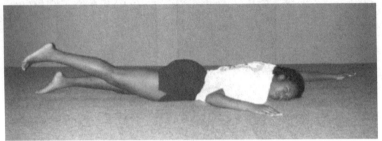

Prone lift – one leg and arm

PRONE LIFT – BOTH LEGS AND ARMS

1. Lie on your stomach with the legs straight, toes pointing downward, and arms straightened above your head;
2. Push your pubic bone into the floor and slowly lift both legs, both arms, and your head until the feet and hands are 3-6 inches from the floor;
3. Hold your legs and arms in this position for 30 seconds;
4. Repeat 3 times. If the third lift is easy, increase the time held by 10 seconds;
5. Do this exercise every other day.

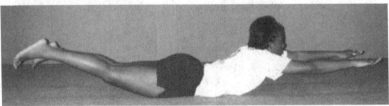

Prone lift – both legs and arms

24

REFERENCES

1. Acasuso-Diaz M, Cisnal A, Collantes-Estevez E. *Quantification of joint laxity: the non-dominant (Spanish) modification (letter)*. British Journal of Rheumatology 34:795-96. 1995.

POSTURE NOTES

POSTURE NOTES (cont.)

LOWER EXTREMITY NOTES

Chapter 3: LOWER EXTREMITY DIAGNOSIS AND TREATMENT

Diagnosis of Lower Extremity Somatic Dysfunction:

1. Lower extremity screening – p.30
2. Lower extremity palpation – pp.31-32
3. Motion testing – integrated into OMT and:
   Hip – p.34
   Knee – p.41
   Ankle – p.47
4. Somatic dysfunction diagnosis – p.33
5. Orthopedic exam as indicated
6. Neurologic exam as indicated

Treatment of Lower Extremity Somatic Dysfunction:

1. OMT

Lower extremity facilitated oscillatory release – p.35
Lateral trochanter counterstrain – p.36
Hip myofascial release – p.37
Hip/pelvis percussion vibrator – p.38
Hip muscle energy – pp.39-40
Patella tendon counterstrain – p.42
Medial meniscus counterstrain – p.43
Knee myofascial release – p.44
Knee percussion vibrator – p.45
Knee articulatory – p.46
Extension ankle counterstrain – p.48
Lateral ankle counterstrain – p.49
Medial ankle counterstrain – p.50

Ankle myofascial release – p.51
Ankle muscle energy – p.52
Ankle thrust – p.53
Interosseous membrane myofascial release – p.54
Fibular head muscle energy – p.55
Calcaneus counterstrain – p.56
Forefoot myofascial release – p.57
Foot articulatory – p.58
Tarsal thrust – p.59
Interphalangeal articulatory – p.60

2. Exercises

Hamstring position of ease – p.61
Hamstring stretch – p.61
Hip abductor position of ease – p.62
Hip abductor stretch – p.62
Medial meniscus position of ease – p.63

Patella position of ease – p.64
Patella mobilization – p.64
Achilles position of ease – p.65
Achilles stretch – p.65
Lateral ankle position of ease – p.66

3. Stabilization

Arch supports
Foot orthotics
Elastic wraps for instability
Joint braces for severe instability

4. Thermal therapy

Heat 20-30 minutes 4-6 times a day for tension or stiffness
Cold 15-20 minutes 4-6 times a day for pain relief

LOWER EXTREMITY ROTATION SCREENING

1. With the patient supine grasp the feet and test external and internal rotation, comparing sides to identify a restriction;
2. If restricted evaluate knee and hip motion.

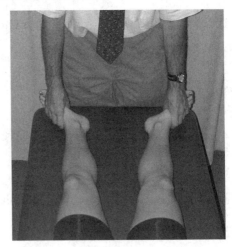

Lower extremity rotation screening

HIP JOINT SCREENING (Fabere test, Patrick maneuver)

1. With the patient supine passively flex the hip and knee to 90°;
2. Holding the knee with one hand and the ankle with your other hand, abduct and externally rotate the hip to its restrictive barriers;
3. Maintain the abduction and external rotation barriers as you extend the leg fully;
4. Compare to the other hip to determine restricted motion;
5. Reproduction of hip or pelvic pain suggests hip joint or sacroiliac arthralgia.

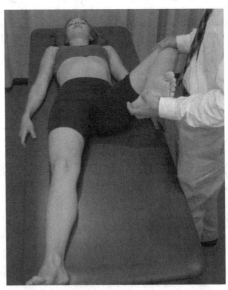

Hip joint screening (Fabere test, Patrick maneuver)

LOWER EXTREMITY PALPATION

1. Palpate the lower extremity for tenderness, tension, and edema at the following locations (see figures p.32):

   1) Greater trochanter – **lateral trochanter tender point** can be on the trochanter or inferior to it in the iliotibial band;
   2) Tibial tuberosity – inferior to patella;
   3) **Patella tendon tender point** – superior to tibial tuberosity and inferior to patella;
   4) **Medial meniscus tender point** – on tibial plateau medial to middle of patella;
   5) **Medial ankle tender point** – ligaments inferior and anterior to medial malleolus;
   6) Metatarsal heads – dorsal foot at distal arch;
   7) Fibular head – inferior and posterior to lateral knee joint;
   8) **Extension ankle tender point** – medial or lateral insertion of gastrocnemius muscle;
   9) **Lateral ankle tender point** – ligaments inferior and anterior to lateral malleolus;
   10) **Calcaneus tender point** – inferior and anterior aspect of heel;
   11) Navicular bone – medial side of plantar foot distal to calcaneus;
   12) Cuboid bone – lateral side of plantar foot distal to calcaneus.

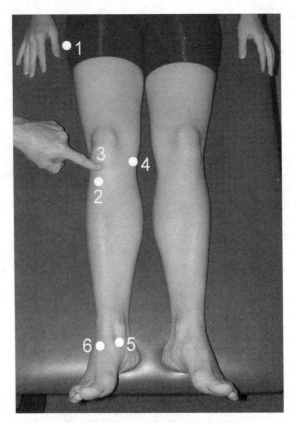

Lower extremity anteromedial palpation

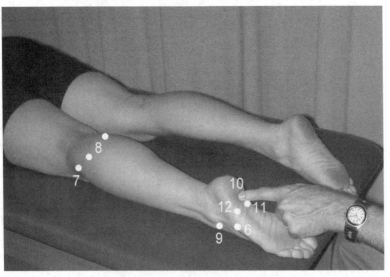

Lower extremity posterolateral palpation

LOWER EXTREMITY SOMATIC DYSFUNCTION

Somatic Dysfunction[1] (position of laxity)	Palpatory Findings	Restriction
Metarsal inferior glide	Tarsal-metatarsal tenderness	Metatarsal superior glide
Metarsal superior glide	Tarsal-metatarsal tenderness	Metatarsal inferior glide
Navicular inversion	Flat foot Navicular tenderness	Navicular eversion
Cuboid inversion	Flat foot Cuboid tenderness	Cuboid eversion
Talus anterior (relative to tibia)	Gastrocnemius tension and tenderness	Ankle dorsiflexion
Talus posterior (relative to tibia)	Tibialis anterior tension and tenderness	Ankle plantar flexion
Fibular head posterior	Fibular head tenderness	Ankle dorsiflexion Fibular head anterolateral glide
Fibular head anterior	Fibular head tenderness	Ankle plantar flexion Fibular head posteromedial glide
Interosseous torsion	Tibialis anterior tension and tenderness	Interosseous torsion
Tibia external rotation	Tibial tuberosity lateral Knee joint or patellar tendon tenderness	Tibia internal rotation
Tibia internal rotation	Tibial tuberosity medial Knee joint or patellar tendon tenderness	Tibia external rotation
Hip abduction	Greater trochanter or iliotibial band tenderness Gluteus tension or tenderness	Hip adduction
Hip adduction	Hip adductor tension or tenderness	Hip abduction
Hip extension	Hamstring or gluteal tension or tenderness	Hip flexion
Hip flexion	Quadriceps or iliopsoas tension or tenderness	Hip extension
Hip external rotation	Gluteal or piriformis tension or tenderness	Hip internal rotation (posterior glide)
Hip internal rotation	Hip adductor tension or tenderness	Hip external rotation (anterior glide)

[1]Somatic dysfunction is described by direction of freer motion but can also be defined by position of a body part or direction of restricted motion.[1]

HIP RANGE OF MOTION

With the patient supine test hip range of motion for each plane of the involved hip and compare to the other side (see HIP MUSCLE ENERGY pp.39-40 for additional illustrations):

1) Abduction – grasp the ankle and move the leg laterally to the abduction barrier;
2) Adduction – grasp the ankle and move the leg medially over the other leg to the adduction barrier;
3) Flexion – palpate the opposite anterior superior iliac spine (ASIS) with one hand, grasp the ankle with the other hand and lift the straightened leg to the flexion barrier which occurs when the opposite ASIS starts to move;
4) Extension – have the patient pull the opposite knee toward the chest and allow the involved leg to hang off the table into the extension barrier which should normally be with the thigh resting on the table;
5) External rotation – flex the hip and knee 90°, hold the knee and ankle and move the knee laterally to the external rotation barrier;
6) Internal rotation – flex the hip and knee 90°, hold the knee and ankle and move the knee medially to the internal rotation barrier.

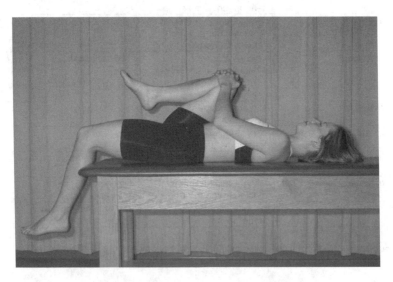

Restricted left hip extension (Thomas test)

LOWER EXTREMITY FACILITATED OSCILLATORY RELEASE

Indication: Lower extremity somatic dysfunction associated with back pain, pelvic pain, leg pain, gait abnormality, or other problems.

Relative contraindications: Acute fracture, deep venous thrombosis, significant patient guarding.

Technique (supine):

1. Standing at the foot of the table, grasp the ankle with one or both hands and lift the leg;
2. Internally rotate the leg and lean backward to stretch the fascia of the lower extremity, adjusting the vector of traction to localize restriction;
3. Initiate oscillatory motion of the leg in a horizontal plane by rhythmically moving your arms left and right, feeling for restricted mobility;
4. Continue lower extremity oscillation or modify its traction and force until you feel mobility improve.

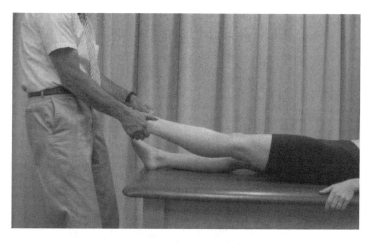

Lower extremity facilitated oscillatory release

LATERAL TROCHANTER COUNTERSTRAIN

Indication: Lateral trochanter tender point associated with hip pain, back pain, leg pain, gait abnormality, and other problems.

Relative contraindications: Deep venous thrombosis.

Technique (supine):

1. Hold the ankle with one hand and locate the tender point on the lateral thigh between the greater trochanter and knee, labeling it 10/10;
2. Abduct and slightly external rotate the leg and retest for tenderness;
3. Fine tune this position with slightly more abduction or external rotation until tenderness is 2/10 or less;
4. Hold this position for 90 seconds while keeping the finger on the tender point;
5. Slowly and passively return the leg to neutral and retest for tenderness.

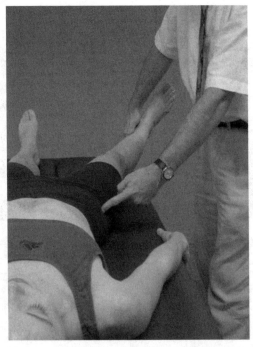

Lateral trochanter counterstrain

Indications: Restricted hip motion related to hip pain, low back pain, pelvic pain, gait abnormality, and other problems.

Relative contraindications: Acute hip fracture or dislocation, deep venous thrombosis, severe hip or knee osteoarthritis.

Technique (supine):

1. Flex the hip and knee to 90° and test internal rotation and external rotation to determine direction of laxity and restriction;
2. Indirect: Move the hip to its position of laxity, apply compression or traction along the femur to facilitate laxity, and follow any tissue release until completed;
3. Direct: Move the hip into its restriction and apply gentle force until tissue give is completed;
4. Retest hip internal and external rotation;
5. Alternative technique: Test flexion-extension, abduction-adduction, and internal-external rotation, stacking the positions of laxity or restriction and performing indirect or direct myofascial release.

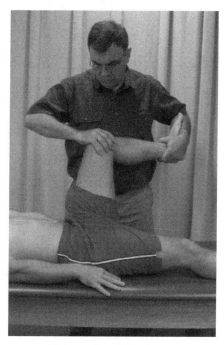

Hip myofascial release

HIP/PELVIS PERCUSSION VIBRATOR

Indications: Restricted hip or pelvis motion associated with hip pain, pelvic pain, back pain, gait abnormality, or other problems.

Relative contraindications: Acute hip fracture or sprain, hip joint inflammation, deep venous thrombosis, lower extremity or pelvic cancer, hip replacement, pregnancy.

Technique (supine):

1. Place your right hand over the left greater trochanter;
2. Place the vibrating percussion pad lightly on the left greater trochanter, avoiding pad bouncing;
3. Alter pad speed, pressure, and angle until vibrations are palpated as strong by the monitoring hand;
4. Maintain contact until the force and rhythm of vibrations return to that of normal tissue;
5. Alternative technique:
   a) Allow the monitoring hand to be pulled toward the pad, resisting any other direction of hand pull;
   b) Maintain percussion until the monitoring hand is pushed away from the pad;
6. Slowly release the monitoring hand and the percussion vibrator and retest motion.

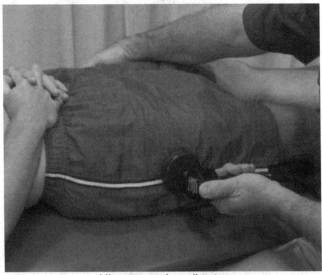

Hip percussion vibrator

Indications: Restricted hip motion related to hip pain, low back pain, pelvic pain, gait abnormality, and other problems.

Relative contraindications: Acute hip fracture or dislocation, acute hip sprain, hip joint inflammation, femoral head avascular necrosis.

Technique (supine):

1. Test hip flexion-extension, abduction-adduction, and internal-external rotation to identify restrictions;
2. Move the hip to its restrictive barrier and ask the patient to gently push the leg away from the restriction against your equal resistance for 3-5 seconds;
3. Slowly move the hip to a new restrictive barrier;
4. Repeat 3-5 times or until motion returns;
5. Retest hip motion.

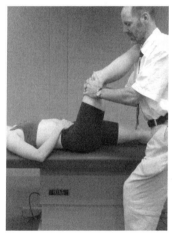

Flexion

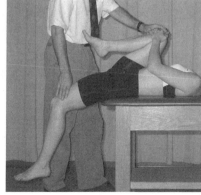

Extension

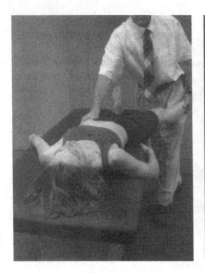
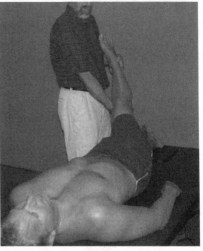

Abduction   Abduction

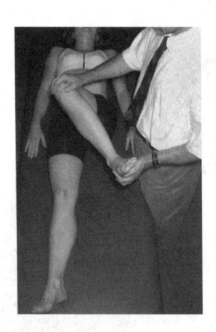

Internal rotation (external rotation opposite)

TIBIAL TORSION PALPATION

1. With the patient supine, place your thumb and index finger of one hand on the lateral margins of the patella;
2. Place the tip of your other index finger on the midline of the tibial tuberosity which should normally be below the middle of the patella;
3. Tibial tuberosity lateral = tibia external rotation;
   Tibial tuberosity medial = tibia internal rotation.

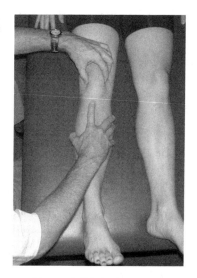

Normal tibial alignment

PATELLA TENDON COUNTERSTRAIN

Indications: Patella tendon tender point associated with knee pain, leg pain, gait abnormality, and other problems.

Relative contraindications: Acute knee sprain with internal derangement, acute patella fracture, deep venous thrombosis.

Technique (supine):

1. Place a pillow or your knee under the foot and locate the tender point in the patella tendon, labeling it 10/10;
2. Push the distal femur posterior to extend the knee and retest for tenderness;
3. Fine tune this position with slight tibia internal or external rotation until tenderness is 2/10 or less;
4. Hold this position for 90 seconds while keeping a finger on the tender point;
5. Slowly and passively return the leg to neutral and retest for tenderness.

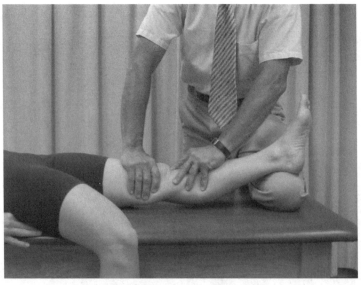

Patella tendon counterstrain

MEDIAL MENISCUS COUNTERSTRAIN

Indications: Medial meniscus tender point associated with knee pain, leg pain, gait abnormality, and other problems.

Relative contraindications: Acute knee sprain with internal derangement, deep venous thrombosis.

Technique (supine):

1. Locate the tender point at the medial knee joint line, labeling it 10/10;
2. Hold the ankle, flex the knee about 60° by dropping the leg off the table, and retest for tenderness;
3. Fine tune this position with slight tibia internal rotation and adduction until tenderness is 2/10 or less;
4. Hold this position for 90 seconds while keeping a finger on the tender point;
5. Slowly and passively return the leg to neutral and retest for tenderness.

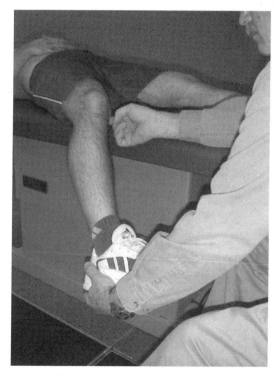

Medial meniscus counterstrain

KNEE MYOFASCIAL RELEASE

Indication: Restricted knee flexion or extension related to knee pain, leg pain, gait abnormality, and other problems.

Relative contraindications: Acute fracture, deep venous thrombosis.

Technique (supine or seated):

1. Grasp the proximal leg with your thumbs on the tibial plateau and hold the foot between your elbow and hip (supine) or between your knees (seated);
2. Move the tibia into anterior-posterior glide, medial-lateral glide, and internal-external rotation to determine directions of laxity and restriction;
3. Indirect: Slowly move the tibia to its positions of laxity and follow any tissue release until completed;
4. Direct: Slowly move the tibia into its restrictions and maintain constant force until tissue give is completed;
5. Retest tibial or knee motion.

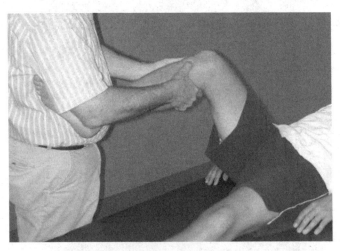

Knee myofascial release

KNEE PERCUSSION VIBRATOR

Indications: Restricted knee or fibular head motion associated with knee pain, knee restriction, gait abnormality, or other problems.

Relative contraindications: Acute knee sprain, knee joint inflammation, deep venous thrombosis, lower extremity cancer, post-knee surgery, knee replacement.

Technique (supine, prone, seated):

1. Place your monitoring hand over the medial knee;
2. Place the vibrating percussion pad lightly on the lateral knee at the distal femur or the fibular head, avoiding pad bouncing;
3. Alter pad speed, pressure, and angle until vibrations are palpated as strong by the monitoring hand;
4. Maintain contact until the force and rhythm of vibrations returns to that of normal tissue;
5. Alternative technique:
   a) Allow the monitoring hand to be pulled toward the pad, resisting any other direction of hand pull;
   b) Maintain percussion until the monitoring hand is pushed away from the pad;
6. Slowly release the monitoring hand and the percussion vibrator and retest motion.

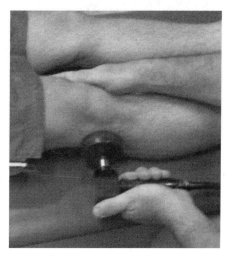

Knee percussion vibrator

KNEE ARTICULATORY

Indication: Restricted tibia internal or external rotation related to knee pain, gait abnormality, and other problems.

Relative contraindications: Joint inflammation, acute sprain, acute fracture, joint hypermobility, deep venous thrombosis, lower extremity cancer, severe knee osteoarthritis.

Technique (supine):

1. Lift the distal femur with one hand to slightly flex the knee;
2. Hold the anterior tibia below the tibial tuberosity with your other hand;
3. In one smooth motion, slowly flex the knee, rotate the tibia into its restriction, and extend the knee;
4. Repeat 3-5 times or until joint mobility returns;
5. Retest tibial rotation.

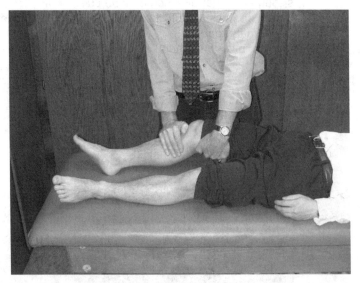

Articulatory for restricted knee internal rotation

ANKLE MOTION

1. With the patient supine or seated induce dorsiflexion and plantar flexion, comparing range for right and left ankles;
2. Restricted dorsiflexion = anterior talus;
   Restricted plantar flexion = posterior talus.

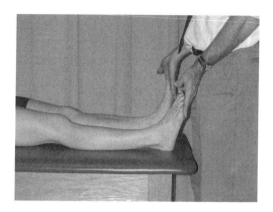

Left ankle restricted dorsiflexion

ANKLE SWING TEST

1. With the patient seated, grasp the feet with your thumbs on the anterior talus;
2. Push the feet posteriorly while holding them horizontal to glide the talus posteriorly and dorsiflex the ankles, comparing sides for restricted motion;
3. Positive swing test = restricted posterior talus glide = anterior talus = plantar flexion somatic dysfunction.

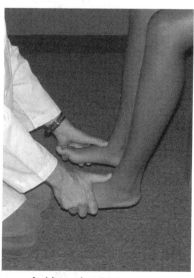

Ankle swing test

EXTENSION ANKLE COUNTERSTRAIN

Indication: Tender point in gastrocnemius muscle associated with ankle pain, leg pain, foot pain, gait abnormality, and other problems.

Relative contraindications: Acute ankle sprain with joint instability, acute fracture, deep venous thrombosis.

Technique (prone):

1. Locate the tender point in the proximal gastrocnemius muscle near its medial or lateral origin, labeling it 10/10;
2. Flex the patient's knee, place your foot on the table, rest the patient's foot on your thigh, and retest for tenderness;
3. Fine tune this position by pushing the patient's foot into your thigh and shifting your thigh position until tenderness is 2/10 or less;
4. Hold this position for 90 seconds while keeping a finger on the tender point;
5. Slowly and passively return the leg to neutral and retest for tenderness.

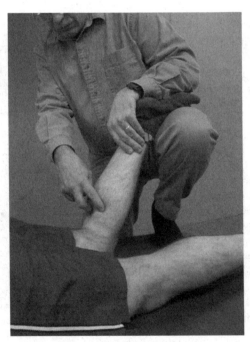

Extension ankle counterstrain

LATERAL ANKLE COUNTERSTRAIN

Indication: Lateral ankle tender point associated with ankle pain, leg pain, foot pain, gait abnormality, and other problems.

Relative contraindications: Acute ankle sprain with joint instability, acute fracture, deep venous thrombosis.

Technique (lateral):

1. With the patient lying on the side of the problem, use one hand to hold the distal tibia and locate the tender point anterior and inferior to the lateral malleolus, labeling it 10/10;
2. Hold the calcaneus with your other hand, evert the foot by pushing the calcaneus toward the floor, and retest for tenderness;
3. Fine tune this position with slightly more or less eversion until tenderness is 2/10 or less;
4. Hold this position for 90 seconds while keeping a finger on the tender point;
5. Slowly and passively return the foot to neutral and retest for tenderness.

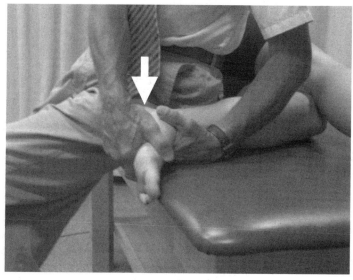

Lateral ankle counterstrain

MEDIAL ANKLE COUNTERSTRAIN

Indication: Medial ankle tender point associated with ankle pain, leg pain, foot pain, gait abnormality, and other problems.

Relative contraindications: Acute ankle sprain with joint instability, acute fracture, deep venous thrombosis.

Technique (lateral):

1. With the patient lying on the opposite side of the problem, use one hand to hold the distal tibia and locate the tender point inferior to the medial malleolus, labeling it 10/10;
2. Invert the foot with your other hand and retest for tenderness;
3. Fine tune this position with slight foot internal rotation and inversion until tenderness is 2/10 or less;
4. Hold this position for 90 seconds while keeping a finger on the tender point;
5. Slowly and passively return the foot to neutral and retest for tenderness.

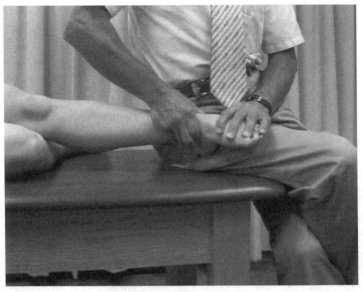

Medial ankle counterstrain

50

ANKLE MYOFASCIAL RELEASE

Indications: Restricted ankle motion related to ankle pain, leg pain, foot pain, gait abnormality, and other problems.

Relative contraindications: Acute fracture or dislocation, calf deep venous thrombosis, acute sprain (direct).

Technique (seated or supine):

1. Hold the calcaneus and plantar surface of the foot with one hand and distal leg with your other hand;
2. Test ankle dorsiflexion and plantar flexion, comparing to the other side to determine directions of laxity and restriction;
3. Indirect: Gently and slowly move the ankle to its position of laxity, apply compression or traction between your hands to facilitate laxity, and follow any tissue release until it is completed;
4. Direct (contraindicated for acute sprain): Slowly move the ankle into its restriction and apply steady force until tissue give is completed;
5. Slowly return the ankle to neutral and retest motion.

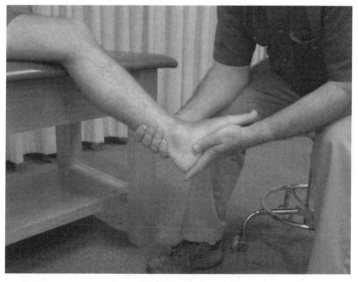

Ankle myofascial release

ANKLE MUSCLE ENERGY

Indications: Restricted ankle motion related to ankle pain, leg pain, foot pain, gait abnormality, and other problems.

Relative contraindications: Acute fracture or dislocation, acute sprain, ankle joint inflammation, calf deep venous thrombosis.

Technique (seated or supine):

1. Test ankle dorsiflexion and plantar flexion, comparing both sides to identify a restriction;
2. Move the ankle to its restrictive barrier and ask the patient to gently push or pull the foot away from the restriction against your equal resistance for 3-5 seconds;
3. Slowly move the ankle to a new restrictive barrier;
4. Repeat 3-5 times or until motion returns;
5. Retest ankle motion.

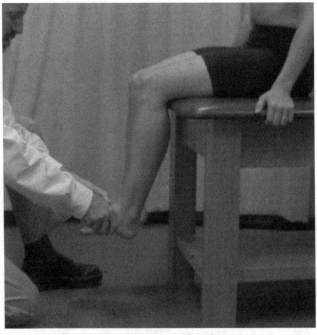

Muscle energy for ankle dorsiflexion restriction

ANKLE THRUST

Indications: Restricted ankle dorsiflexion related to ankle pain, leg pain, foot pain, gait abnormality, and other problems.

Relative contraindications: Acute fracture or dislocation, acute sprain, ankle joint inflammation, ankle joint hypermobility, calf deep venous thrombosis.

Technique (supine):

1. Stand at the foot of the table and grasp the foot with your fifth fingers on the dorsal talus and thumbs on the plantar surface near the distal metatarsal heads;
2. Evert the foot and move the ankle to its dorsiflexion restrictive barrier;
3. Ask the patient to take a deep breath and during exhalation apply a short and quick caudad tug of the foot while maintaining the dorsiflexion barrier;
4. Retest ankle dorsiflexion.

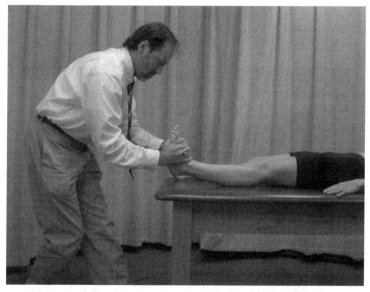

Thrust for ankle dorsiflexion restriction

INTEROSSEOUS MEMBRANE MYOFASCIAL RELEASE

Indication: Restricted leg fascial rotation related to leg pain, ankle pain, gait abnormality, and other problems. The technique can be adapted for restricted forearm fascia rotation related arm pain and other problems.

Relative contraindications: Acute sprain, acute fracture, deep venous thrombosis.

Technique (supine):

1. Hold the proximal leg at the tibial tuberosity and fibular head with one hand and the distal leg at the lateral and medial malleoli with your other hand;
2. Rotate the hands in opposite directions and then reverse directions to determine torsional laxity versus restriction;
3. Indirect: Use both hands to slowly rotate the lower leg into its position of torsional laxity, apply compression or traction between your hands to facilitate laxity, and follow any tissue release until completed;
4. Direct: Use both hands to slowly rotate the lower leg into its torsional restriction and apply steady force until tissue give is completed;
5. Retest rotational torsion.

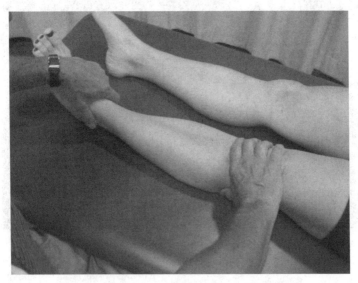

Interosseous membrane myofascial release

FIBULAR HEAD MOTION

1. With the patient supine and knees bent, place your thumb and index finger on the anterior and posterior sides of the proximal fibular head;
2. Pull the fibular head anterolaterally and push it posteromedially to identify joint glide;
3. Restricted anterolateral glide = posterior fibular head;
   Restricted posteromedial glide = anterior fibular head.

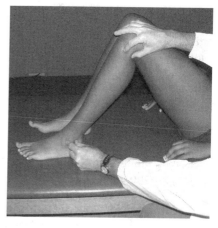

Fibular head motion

FIBULAR HEAD MUSCLE ENERGY

Indication: Posterior fibular head associated with knee pain, ankle pain, gait abnormality, and other problems.

Relative contraindications: Acute ankle sprain, acute fibular fracture, deep venous thrombosis, ankle joint laxity.

Technique (supine or seated):

1. Flex the knee about 40°;
2. Pull the fibular head antero-laterally while dorsiflexing the foot to its restrictive barrier;
3. Ask the patient to plantar flex the foot against your equal resistance for 3-5 seconds;

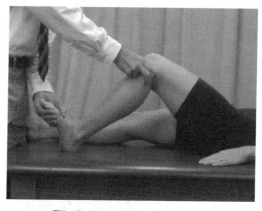

Fibular head muscle energy

4. Slowly move the ankle to a new dorsiflexion barrier as you continue pulling the fibular head anterolaterally;
5. Repeat 3-5 times or until fibular head mobility returns;
6. Retest fibular head motion;
7. For an anterior fibular head reverse all directions in steps 2-4.

CALCANEUS COUNTERSTRAIN

Indication: Calcaneus tender point associated with foot pain, ankle pain, gait abnormality, and other problems.

Relative contraindications: Acute ankle sprain with joint instability, acute fracture, deep venous thrombosis.

Technique (prone):

1. Locate the tender point on the bottom of the foot at the distal edge of the calcaneus, labeling it 10/10;
2. Flex the patient's knee, place your foot on the table, rest the patient's foot on your thigh, and retest for tenderness;
3. Fine tune this position by pushing the patient's leg into your thigh, shifting your thigh position, and slightly inverting or everting the foot until tenderness is 2/10 or less;
4. Hold this position for 90 seconds while keeping a finger on the tender point;
5. Slowly and passively return the foot to neutral and retest for tenderness.

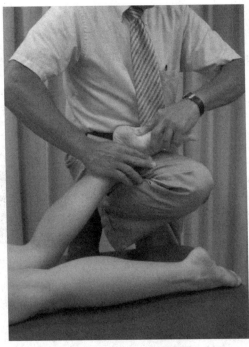

Calcaneus counterstrain

Indications: Restricted forefoot inversion or eversion related to foot pain, ankle pain, gait abnormality, and other problems.

Relative contraindications: Acute fracture or dislocation.

Technique (seated or supine):

1. Hold the calcaneus firmly with one hand and the forefoot with your other hand at the level of the proximal tarsal-metatarsal joints;
2. Test forefoot inversion and eversion to determine directions of ease and restriction, comparing to the other foot if needed;
3. Indirect: Gently and slowly move the forefoot to its position of laxity, apply compression or traction between your hands to facilitate laxity, and follow any tissue release until it is completed;
4. Direct: Slowly move the forefoot into its restriction and apply steady force until tissue give is completed;
5. Slowly return the forefoot to neutral and retest motion.

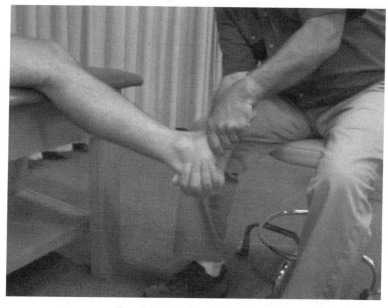

Forefoot myofascial release

FOOT ARTICULATORY

Indication: Metatarsal joint restriction associated with foot pain, ankle pain, gait abnormality, and other problems.

Relative contraindications: Acute fracture or sprain, joint inflammation, joint hypermobility.

Technique (supine):

1. Stabilize the proximal bone of the joint being treated with one hand;
2. Grasp the distal bone with your other hand and gently test superior and inferior glide;
3. If restricted, slowly circumduct the distal bone clockwise and counterclockwise 3-5 times or until motion returns;
4. Retest metatarsal motion.

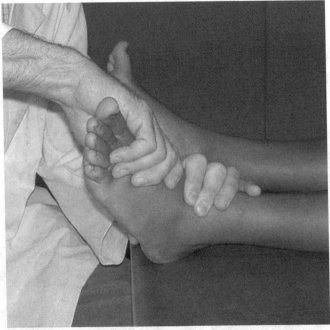

Articulatory for 1st and 2nd tarsal-metatarsal joints

TARSAL THRUST (Hiss whip)

Indication: Navicular or cuboid tenderness and restriction associated with foot pain, ankle pain, gait abnormality, and other problems.

Relative contraindications: Acute fracture or sprain, joint inflammation, joint hypermobility.

Technique (prone):

1. Hold the foot with both thumbs on the medial aspect of the navicular or cuboid bone;
2. Flex the hip and knee by dropping the leg off the table;
3. Plantar flex the ankle and push the tarsal bone to its restrictive barrier:
   Navicular – push dorsally and medially;
   Cuboid – push dorsally and laterally;
4. Apply a short and quick thrust with the thumbs into the restrictive barrier while swinging the ankle into plantar flexion;
5. Retest arch flexibility (tenderness may not be alleviated immediately).

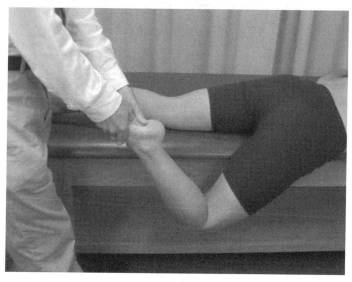

Cuboid thrust

INTERPHALANGEAL ARTICULATORY (foot or hand)

Indication: Interphalangeal restriction associated with foot or hand pain and other related problems.

Relative contraindications: Acute fracture or sprain, joint inflammation, joint hypermobility.

Technique (seated or supine):

1. Stabilize the proximal bone of the joint being treated with one hand;
2. Grasp the distal bone with your other hand and gently flex and extend it to identify motion restriction;
3. Apply traction to the distal bone and slowly circumduct it in both directions 3-5 times or until motion returns;
4. Retest interphalangeal motion.

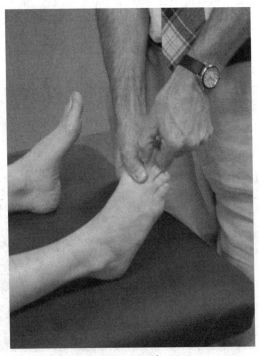

Articulatory for 2nd PIP joint

HAMSTRING POSITION OF EASE

1. Lay face down and place a pillow or two under the ankle of the involved leg;
2. If comfortable, take a few deep breaths and rest in this position for 2-5 minutes;
3. Use this position as often as needed for pain relief.

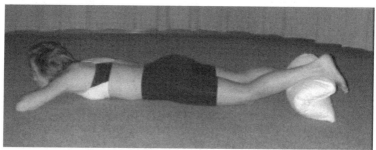

Hamstring position of ease

HAMSTRING STRETCH

1. Sit with one leg straight and the hand on the same side on the floor behind you;
2. Keeping the leg straight, reach with the other hand toward the foot as far as you can comfortably go;
3. Take a few deep breaths and stretch for 10-20 seconds;
4. Repeat for the other leg;
5. Do this stretch 2-4 times a day.

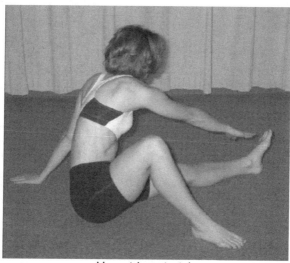

Hamstring stretch

HIP ABDUCTOR POSITION OF EASE

1. Lie on your back with two or three pillows placed next to the painful hip;
2. Bend the knee of the involved leg and allow it to rest on the pillows;
3. If comfortable, take a few deep breaths and rest in this position for 2-5 minutes;
4. Slowly straighten the leg;
5. Repeat 2-4 times a day or as needed for pain relief.

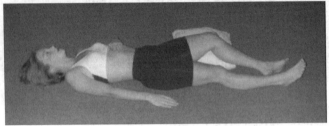

Hip abductor position of ease

HIP ABDUCTOR STRETCH

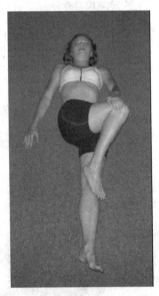

1. Lying on your back, bend one leg up and let it fall across the other leg;
2. Use the opposite arm to grasp the bent leg above the knee and pull it across the other leg as far as it will comfortably go;
3. Take a few deep breaths and stretch for 10-20 seconds;
4. Repeat to the other side;
5. Do this stretch 1-4 times a day.

Hip abductor stretch

MEDIAL MENISCUS POSITION OF EASE

1. Lie on the side of the painful knee;
2. Extend the painful knee backward and rest the end of your foot on a pillow;
3. If comfortable, take a few deep breaths and rest in this position for 2-5 minutes;
4. Use as often as needed for pain relief.

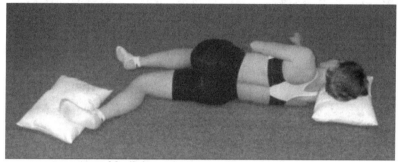

Medial meniscus position of ease

PATELLA POSITION OF EASE

1. Lie on your back with the legs straight;
2. Place a pillow or two under your foot on the side of thigh or knee pain;
3. If comfortable, take a few deep breaths and rest in this position for 2-5 minutes;
4. Use as often as needed for pain relief.

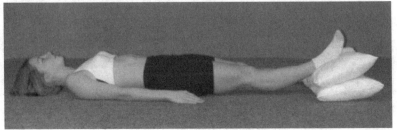

Patella position of ease

PATELLA MOBILIZATION[2]

1. Sit with your legs straight and a hand on the floor behind you;
2. Use the web of your other hand to push the involved kneecap down toward the big toe as far as it will comfortably go;
3. Gently push the lower leg up toward the ceiling until knee pain occurs;
4. Release and repeat 2-5 times;
5. Do this mobilization 2-4 times a day.

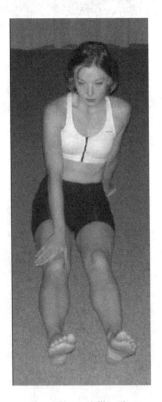

Patella mobilization

ACHILLES/GASTROCNEMIUS POSITION OF EASE

1. Lay face down with the involved foot resting on a pillow or two;
2. If comfortable, take a few deep breaths and rest in this position for 2-5 minutes;
3. Repeat 2-4 times a day or as needed for pain relief.

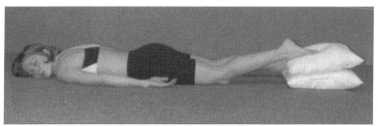

Achilles/gastrocnemius position of ease

ACHILLES/GASTROCNEMIUS STRETCH

1. Stand 3-4 feet from a wall;
2. Step toward the wall with one leg, placing your hands on the wall;
3. Keep the heel of your back leg on the floor and slowly lean into the wall until you feel a stretch at the back of the leg;
4. Take a few deep breaths and stretch for 10-20 seconds;
5. Repeat this stretch with the involved knee slightly bent;
6. Repeat for the other leg;
7. Do these stretches 2-4 times a day.

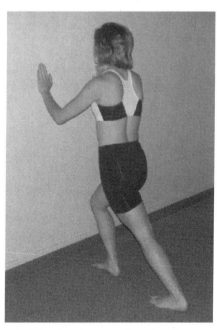

Achilles/gastrocnemius stretch

LATERAL ANKLE POSITION OF EASE

1. Lie on the side of ankle pain with a pillow under your leg and the foot hanging off the end of the pillow;
2. If comfortable, take a few deep breaths and rest in this position for 2-5 minutes;
3. Repeat 2-4 times a day or as needed for pain relief.

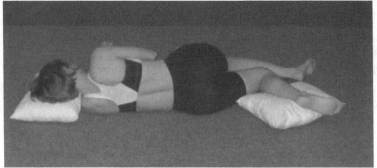

Lateral ankle position of ease

REFERENCES

1. Glossary of Osteopathic Terminology, p.1249 in Ward RC, Ed. *Foundations for Osteopathic Medicine, 2nd Edition.* Lippincott Williams & Wilkins, Philadelphia, 2003.

2. Baycroft CM. *A self-treatment method for patello-femoral dysfunction.* Journal of Manual Medicine 5:25-26. 1990.

LOWER EXTREMITY NOTES

Chapter 4: PELVIC DIAGNOSIS AND TREATMENT

Diagnosis of Pelvis Somatic Dysfunction

1. Screening tests
   Standing flexion test – p.72
   ASIS compression test – p.72
2. Palpation – pp.73-76
3. Pelvis somatic dysfunction – p.77

Treatment of Pelvis Somatic Dysfunction

1. OMT

   Iliopsoas counterstrain – p.78
   Lumbosacral myofascial release – p.79
   Pelvis percussion vibrator – p.80
   Hip/pelvis percussion vibrator – see p.38
   Anterior innominate muscle energy – p.81
   Anterior innominate thrust, lateral recumbent – p.82
   Anterior innominate thrust, supine – p.83
   Posterior innominate muscle energy – p.84
   Posterior innominate thrust, lateral recumbent – p.85
   Posterior innominate thrust, supine – p.86
   Superior innominate shear thrust – p.86
   Pubic muscle energy/thrust – pp.87-88
   Sacroiliac articulatory – p.89

2. Exercises

   Iliopsoas position of ease – p.90
   Iliopsoas stretch – p.90
   Quadriceps position of ease – p.91
   Quadriceps stretch – p.91
   Pubic mobilization – p.92

3. Thermal therapy

   Heat 20-30 minutes 4-6 times a day for tension or stiffness
   Cold 15-20 minutes 4-6 times a day for pain relief

4. Stabilization

   Lumbosacral support belt for overuse strain
   Prolotherapy for ligament laxity and joint hypermobility

STANDING FLEXION TEST

1. Place your thumbs on the undersurface of the posterior superior iliac spines (PSIS) of the standing patient;
2. Ask the patient to bend forward with the legs straight and allow your thumbs to follow PSIS movement;
3. The side of last superior PSIS movement is the side of pelvis restriction;
4. False positives: Contralateral hamstring tightness; Short leg; Sacral somatic dysfunction on same side.

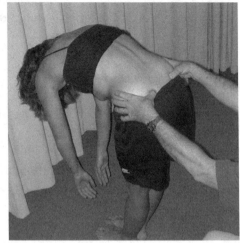

Standing flexion test

ASIS COMPRESSION TEST

1. With the patient supine, place your palms on the anterior superior iliac spines (ASIS);
2. Push posteromedially on one ASIS while monitoring the other ASIS and repeat for the opposite side;
3. Resistance to posteromedial pressure indicates sacroiliac joint restriction on that side.

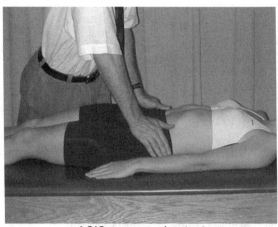

ASIS compression test

PELVIS PALPATION – ANTERIOR

1. Palpate for tenderness at the following locations:

    a) **Iliacus tender point** – 1" medial and slightly inferior to ASIS;
    b) Pubic symphysis – anterior surface.

2. Palpate for symmetry at the following locations after seating the pelvis:

    a) Seating the pelvis: Have the supine patient bend the knees, place the feet on the table, lift the pelvis off the table and set it down, and straighten the legs;
    b) ASIS levelness – place your thumbs on the undersurface of the ASIS and compare for superior-inferior levelness, naming for the side of pelvis restriction;
    c) Pubic tubercle levelness – place your thumbs on the superior surface of the pubic tubercles located 1/4-1/2" lateral to the symphysis and compare for superior-inferior levelness, naming for the side of pelvis restriction.

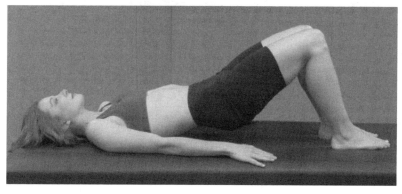

Seating the pelvis before anterior palpation

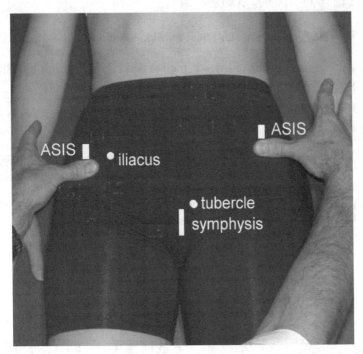

Anterior pelvis palpation (ASIS asymmetry shown)

PELVIS PALPATION – POSTERIOR

1. Palpate for tender points at the following locations:

   a) **Piriformis** – musculature halfway between greater
      trochanter and middle of sacrum.

2. Palpate for symmetry at the following locations after seating the
   pelvis:

   a) Seating the pelvis: With the patient prone lift the legs to flex
      the knees as far as they will comfortably go and then return
      the legs to the table;
   b) PSIS levelness – place your thumbs on the undersurface of
      the PSIS and compare for superior-inferior levelness,
      naming for the side of pelvis restriction.

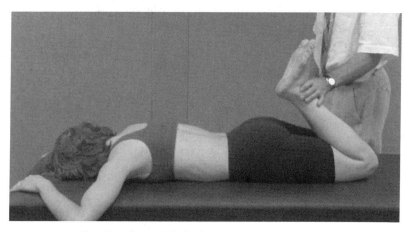

Seating the pelvis before posterior palpation

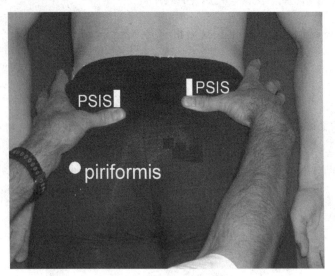

Posterior pelvis palpation (PSIS asymmetry shown)

PELVIC SOMATIC DYSFUNCTION

POSITIONAL DIAGNOSIS	ASIS	PSIS	Pubic Symphysis	Pubic Tubercle
Anterior innominate	inferior	superior	–	–
Posterior innominate	superior	inferior	–	–
Superior innominate shear	superior	superior	–	–
Inferior innominate shear	inferior	inferior	–	–
Pubic compression	–	–	tender	symmetrical
Superior pubic shear	–	–	tender	superior
Inferior pubic shear			tender	inferior

ILIOPSOAS COUNTERSTRAIN

Indication: Iliacus or psoas tender point associated with abdominal pain, pelvic pain, back pain, and other problems.

Relative contraindications: Acute lumbar or hip fracture, hip dislocation.

Technique (supine):

1. Stand beside the patient and locate the tender point 1" medial and slightly inferior to the ASIS, labeling it 10/10;
2. Cross the ankles and passively flex the knees and hips 90°, allowing the hips to externally rotate;
3. Retest for tenderness;
4. Fine tune this position with increased hip flexion until tenderness is 2/10 or less;
5. Hold the position of relief for 90 seconds while keeping a finger on the tender point;
6. Slowly and passively return the legs to the table and retest for tenderness.

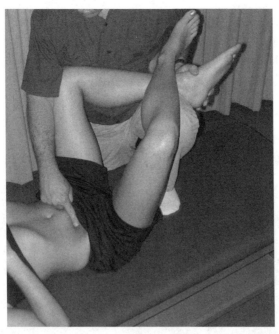

Psoas tender point and counterstrain position

LUMBOSACRAL MYOFASCIAL RELEASE (pelvic diaphragm)

Indication: Restricted lumbosacral fascia rotation related to low back pain, pelvic pain, edema, and other problems.

Relative contraindications: Acute pelvic fracture.

Technique (supine or prone):

1. Place your palms over the lateral pelvis and simultaneously lift one side while pushing the other side posteriorly to induce lumbosacral fascia rotation;
2. Repeat for the other direction to identify rotational restriction and laxity;
3. Indirect: Rotate the lumbosacral fascia to its position of laxity and follow any tissue release until completed;
4. Direct: Rotate the lumbosacral fascia into its restriction and apply steady force until tissue give is completed;
5. Retest lumbosacral fascia rotation.

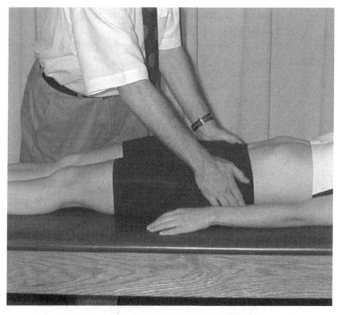

Lumbosacral myofascial release

PELVIS PERCUSSION VIBRATOR

Indications: Restricted pelvis motion associated with hip pain, pelvic pain, back pain, or other problems.

Relative contraindications: Acute pelvis fracture, sacroiliitis, deep venous thrombosis, intrapelvic cancer, recent pelvic surgery, pregnancy.

Technique (lateral):

1. With the patient lying on the non-restricted side with knees and hips flexed, place your monitoring hand over the iliac crest;
2. Place the vibrating percussion pad lightly on the ischial tuberosity, avoiding pad bouncing;
3. Alter pad speed, pressure, and angle until vibrations are palpated as strong by the monitoring hand;
4. Maintain contact until the force and rhythm of vibration returns to that of normal tissue.
5. Alternative technique:
   a) Allow the monitoring hand to be pulled toward the pad, resisting any other direction of hand pull;
   b) Maintain percussion until the monitoring hand is pushed away from the pad;
6. Slowly release the monitoring hand and the percussion vibrator and retest motion.

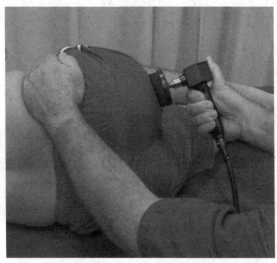

Pelvis percussion vibrator

ANTERIOR INNOMINATE MUSCLE ENERGY

Indication: Anterior innominate rotation or inferior pubic shear associated with back pain, pelvic pain, hip pain, short leg syndrome, and other problems.

Relative contraindications: Acute pelvis fracture, sacroiliac joint inflammation, severe hip arthritis.

Technique (supine):

1. Stand beside the involved side, flex and adduct the hip to its restrictive barrier, and pull the ischial tuberosity anteriorly. For inferior pubic shear push the ischial tuberosity superiorly;
2. Ask the patient to push the knee into your shoulder for 3-5 seconds against your equal resistance;
3. Slowly pull the ischial tuberosity anteriorly and flex the hip to new restrictive barriers;
4. Repeat 3-5 times or until pelvic mobility returns.

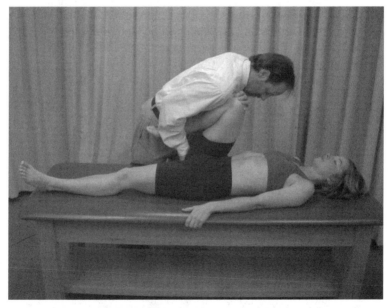

Muscle energy for right anterior innominate

ANTERIOR INNOMINATE THRUST – LATERAL RECUMBENT

Indication: Anterior innominate rotation associated with back pain, hip pain, short leg syndrome, and other problems.

Relative contraindications: Acute lumbar sprain, undiagnosed radiculopathy, acute vertebral fracture, acute herniated or ruptured disc, spondylosis, sacroiliitis, sacroiliac joint hypermobility.

Technique:

1. Stand in front of the patient who is lying with the involved pelvis upward;
2. Flex the involved hip to 90° and drop the leg off the table;
3. Rotate the back toward the table by lifting the table-side arm until you feel rotation at the lumbosacral junction;
4. Use your cephalad arm to stabilize the shoulder, place your other forearm across the ischial tuberosity, and lean over top of that arm;
5. Ask the patient to take a deep breath and during exhalation slowly push the ischial tuberosity toward the femur to take up the rotational slack;
6. At the end of exhalation apply a short quick thrust with your arm and body onto the ischial tuberosity and toward the femur;
7. Recheck sacroiliac mobility or pelvis symmetry.

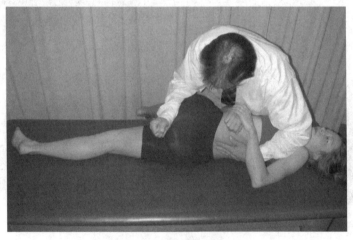

Lateral recumbent thrust for left anterior innominate

Indication: Anterior innominate rotation associated with back pain, pelvis pain, hip pain, short leg syndrome, and other problems.

Relative contraindications: Acute sacroiliac sprain, hip or knee instability, sacroiliac joint hypermobility.

Technique:

1. Stand at the foot of the table and grasp the leg just above the ankle with both hands above the malleoli;
2. Lift the leg to about 30° hip flexion and slightly abduct and internally rotate the leg;
3. Ask the patient to take a deep breath and during exhalation apply a firm and quick caudad tug down the leg;
4. Retest sacroiliac motion or pelvis symmetry.

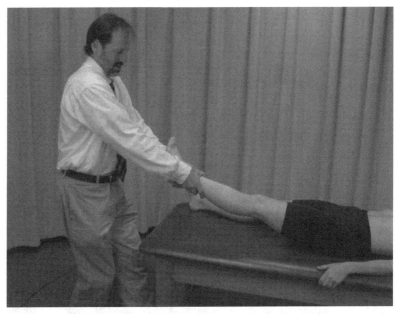

Traction tug for left anterior innominate rotation

POSTERIOR INNOMINATE MUSCLE ENERGY

Indication: Posterior innominate rotation or superior pubic shear associated with back pain, pelvic pain, hip pain, short leg syndrome, and other problems.

Relative contraindications: Acute pelvic fracture, sacroiliac joint inflammation, severe hip arthritis.

Technique (supine):

1. Stand on the involved side and hold the opposite anterior superior iliac spine;
2. Move the involved leg off the table and allow the leg to drop to the hip extension restrictive barrier. For superior pubic shear the ischial tuberosity should remain on the table;
3. Ask the patient to push the thigh upward for 3-5 seconds against your equal resistance;
4. Slowly extend the hip to a new restrictive barrier;
5. Repeat 3-5 times or until pelvic mobility returns.

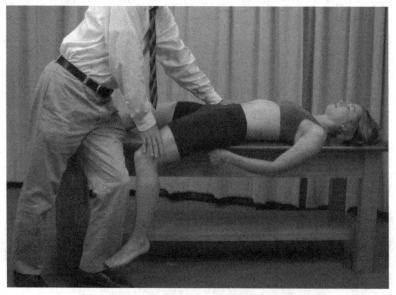

Muscle energy for left posterior innominate

Indication: Posterior innominate rotation associated with back pain, hip pain, short leg syndrome, and other problems.

Relative contraindications: Acute lumbar sprain, undiagnosed radiculopathy, acute vertebral fracture, acute herniated or ruptured disc, sacroiliac joint hypermobility.

Technique:

1. Stand in front of the patient who is lying with the involved pelvis upward;
2. Flex the involved hip until movement is felt at the lumbosacral junction and then tuck that foot behind the other knee;
3. Rotate the back toward the table by lifting the table-side arm until you feel rotation at the lumbosacral junction;
4. Use your cephalad arm to stabilize the shoulder, place your other hand on the posterior aspect of the iliac crest, and lean over top of that hand;
5. Ask the patient to take a deep breath and during exhalation slowly push the iliac crest toward the femur to take up the rotational slack;
6. At the end of exhalation apply a short quick thrust with your arm and body onto the iliac crest toward the femur;
7. Recheck sacroiliac mobility or pelvis symmetry.

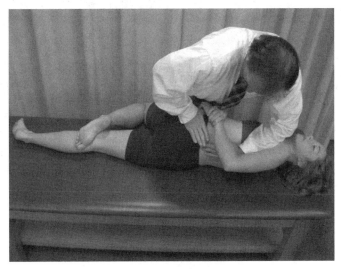

Lateral recumbent thrust for left posterior innominate

POSTERIOR INNOMINATE THRUST – SUPINE

Indication: Posterior innominate rotation or superior innominate shear associated with back pain, pelvis pain, hip pain, and other problems.

Relative contraindications: Acute sacroiliac sprain, sacroiliac joint hypermobility, hip or knee instability.

Technique:

1. Stand at the foot of the table and grasp above the ankle with both hands above the malleoli;
2. Slightly abduct and internally rotate the leg;
3. Ask the patient to take a deep breath and during exhalation apply a firm and quick caudad tug down the leg;
4. Retest sacroiliac motion or pelvis symmetry.

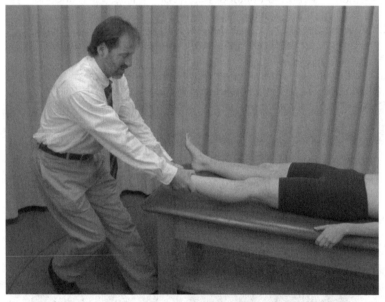

Traction tug for left posterior innominate rotation or superior innominate shear

Indication: Pubic symphysis compression or shear associated with pelvic pain, low back pain, and other problems.

Relative contraindications: Acute pelvis fracture, post-partum.

Technique (supine):

1. Grasp the outside of both knees which are flexed with feet flat on the table;
2. Ask the patient to push the knees apart for 3-5 seconds against your equal resistance;
3. Separate the knees by holding the inside of the knees and ask the patient to push the knees together for 3-5 seconds against your equal resistance;
4. Repeat 3-5 times or until pubic mobilization occurs;
5. If needed, add a thrust to step 3 by applying a short and quick lateral push to overcome adduction contraction and further separate the knees;
6. Retest for pubic asymmetry.

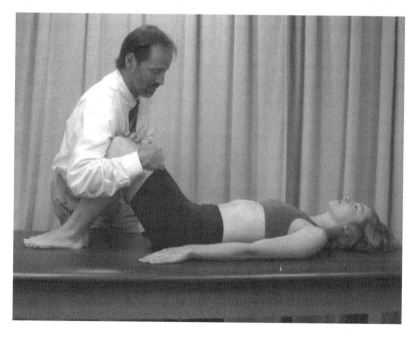

Abduction muscle energy

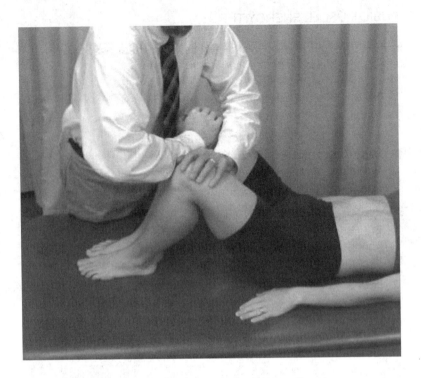

Adduction muscle energy/abduction thrust

SACROILIAC ARTICULATORY

Indication: Sacroiliac joint (SIJ) restriction related to back pain, pelvis pain, hip pain, and other problems.

Relative contraindications: Acute sprain or fracture, SIJ hypermobility, SIJ inflammation, hip arthritis, deep venous thrombosis, premature labor.

Technique (lateral Sims):

1. Stand behind the patient who is lying on the uninvolved side with the chest down;
2. Place the thenar eminence of your cephalad hand on the sacral base of the restricted SIJ and grasp the knee with your other hand;
3. Lean into the sacral base to stabilize the sacrum, have the patient take a deep breath and hold it, and slowly flex the hip to its restrictive barrier;
4. Slowly abduct and externally rotate the hip to its restrictive barrier;
5. Maintain the abduction barrier and slowly extend the hip fully;
6. Repeat as one smooth motion 3-5 times or until joint motion returns;
7. Retest sacroiliac motion.

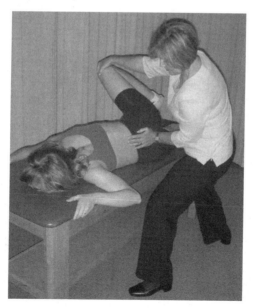

Flexion, abduction, and external rotation

ILIOPSOAS POSITION OF EASE

1. Lie on your back with legs propped up on a chair or stool;
2. Cross your ankles with the foot on the side of back or pelvic pain on top;
3. Let your knees fall apart;
4. If comfortable, take a few deep breaths and rest in this position for 2-5 minutes;
5. Slowly uncross your legs, bring them down, and roll to one side before getting up;
6. Use this position 2-4 times a day or as needed for pain relief.

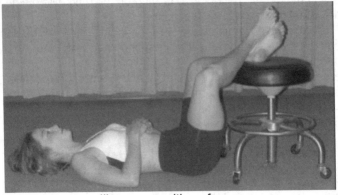

Iliopsoas position of ease

ILIOPSOAS STRETCH[1]

1. Kneel with one foot on the floor a few feet in front of the other knee;
2. Slowly lean forward onto the front leg while using your hand to push the other hip forward over your back leg;
4. Take a few deep breaths and stretch for 10-20 seconds;
5. Repeat to the opposite side;
6. Do this stretch 1-4 times a day.

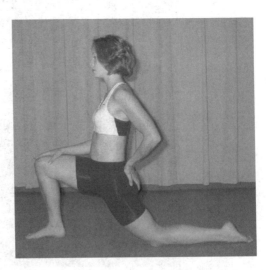

Left iliopsoas stretch

QUADRICEPS POSITION OF EASE

1. Lie on your back with the legs straight;
2. Place a pillow or two under your foot on the side of thigh or knee pain;
3. If comfortable, take a few deep breaths and rest in this position for 2-5 minutes;
4. Use as often as needed for pain relief.

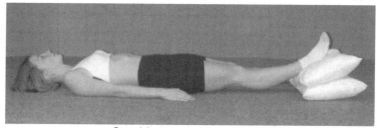

Quadriceps position of ease

QUADRICEPS STRETCH

1. Lie on your back with the involved leg hanging off the end of the bed or table;
2. Pull your other knee toward the chest;
3. Let the foot of the involved leg hang down as far as it will comfortably go;
4. Take a few deep breaths and stretch for 10-20 seconds;
5. Repeat for the other leg;
6. Do this stretch 2-4 times a day.

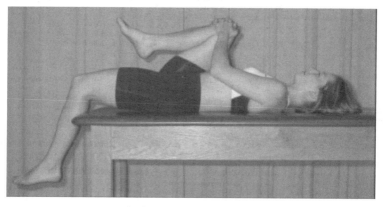

Left quadriceps stretch

PUBIC MOBILIZATION

1. Lie on your back with knees bent, feet on the floor, and head on a pillow or two;
2. Place your hands on the outside of the thighs;
3. Push your knees outward against resistance from your hands for 3-5 seconds;
4. Place a firm ball between the knees;
5. Push your knees inward against the ball for 3-5 seconds;
6. Repeat 1-3 times;
7. Do up to twice a day if helpful.

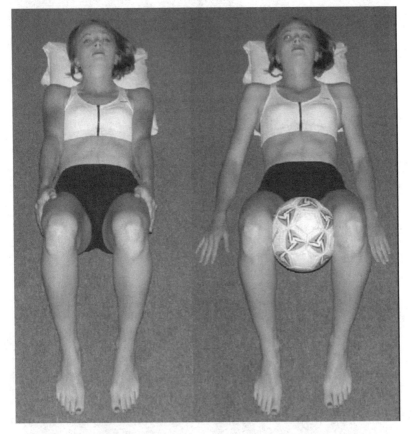

Abduction contraction   Adduction contraction

REFERENCE

1. Adapted from Greenman PE. *Principles of Manual Medicine, 2nd Edition* Williams & Wilkins, Baltimore, 1996.

PELVIS NOTES

PELVIS NOTES (cont.)

SACRAL NOTES

Chapter 5: SACRAL DIAGNOSIS AND TREATMENT

Diagnosis of Sacral Somatic Dysfunction

1. Screening tests
   Seated flexion test – p.98
   ASIS compression test – see p.72
2. Palpation – pp.98-99
3. Sacral motion tests – to determine flexion or extension restriction
   Lumbosacral spring test – p.100
   Backward bending test – p.100
   Respiratory motion test – p.101
4. Sacral somatic dysfunction – pp.102-103

Treatment of Sacral Somatic Dysfunction

1. OMT
   Sacrum counterstrain – p.105
   Mid-pole sacroiliac counterstrain – p.106
   Piriformis counterstrain – p.107
   Sacral rocking/myofascial release – p.108
   Lumbosacral myofascial release – see p.79
   Sacroiliac percussion vibrator – p.109
   Sacrum facilitated oscillatory release – p.110
   Forward sacral torsion muscle energy – p.111
   Backward sacral torsion muscle energy – p.112
   Sacral extension muscle energy – p.113
   Sacral flexion muscle energy – p.114
   Unilateral sacral flexion thrust – p.115
   Sacroiliac articulatory – see p.89

2. Exercises

   Piriformis position of ease – p.116
   Piriformis stretch – p.116
   Sacroiliac mobilization – p.117
   Sacroiliac sidebending mobilization – p.118

3. Thermal therapy

   Heat 20-30 minutes 4-6 times a day for tension or stiffness
   Cold 15-20 minutes 4-6 times a day for pain relief

4. Stabilization

   Lumbosacral support belt for overuse strain
   Prolotherapy for ligament laxity and joint hypermobility

SEATED FLEXION TEST

1. Place your thumbs on the undersurface of the posterior superior iliac spines (PSIS) of the seated patient;
2. Ask the patient to bend forward with feet on the floor and allow your thumbs to follow PSIS movement;
3. The side of last superior PSIS movement is the side of sacrum restriction;
4. False positives: Pelvis somatic dysfunction on same side.

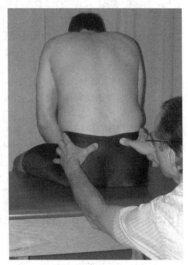

Seated flexion test

SACRAL PALPATION

1. Stand to one side of the prone patient;
2. Palpate for tenderness at the following locations:
   a) **sacrum tender points**
      sacral base on both sides and midline
      middle sacrum on both sides and midline
      lower sacrum on both sides and midline
   b) sacrococcygeal junction;
   c) tip of coccyx;
   d) **mid-pole sacroiliac tender point** - lateral sacrum 1-2" inferior to the PSIS (see p.108);
   e) **piriformis tender point** – halfway between mid-line of sacrum and greater trochanter (see p.109);
3. Sacral base levelness: Place your thumbs on the sacral base just medial to the PSIS and compare for anterior-posterior levelness;
4. Inferior lateral angle (ILA) levelness: Place your thumbs on the posterior surface and compare for anterior-posterior levelness or place your thumbs on the inferior surface and compare for superior-inferior levelness.

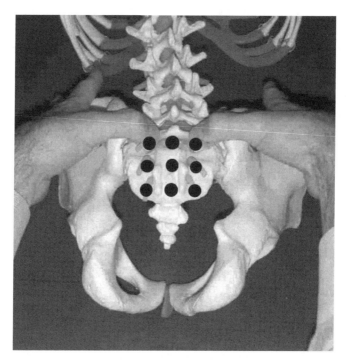

Sacral base palpation (tender points shown)

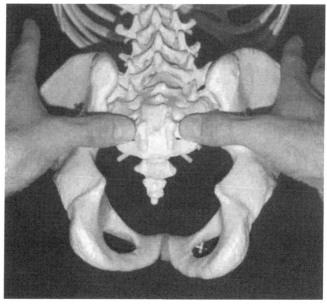

ILA palpation

LUMBOSACRAL SPRING TEST

1. With the patient prone, use one or both palms to firmly push the lumbosacral junction in an anterior direction several times;
2. Ease of motion (negative test) indicates sacral flexion ease, extension restriction;
3. Positive test = resistance to springing = sacral flexion restriction, extension ease.

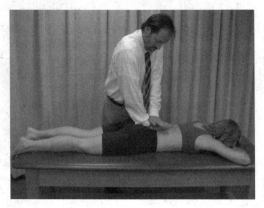

Lumbosacral spring test

BACKWARD BENDING TEST (lumbosacral flexion test)

1. With the patient prone, place your thumbs on each side of the sacral base to identify asymmetry;
2. Ask the patient to place the elbows on the table and lift the upper back to induce relative sacral flexion;
3. Decreased sacral base asymmetry (negative test) indicates sacral flexion ease, extension restriction;
4. Positive test = increased sacral base asymmetry = sacral flexion restriction, extension ease.

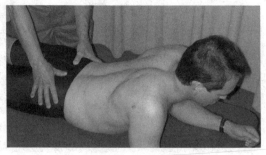

Backward bending test

RESPIRATORY MOTION TESTING

1. With the patient prone, let your hand rest gently on the sacrum with fingertips at sacral base and palm at coccyx;
2. Ask the patient to take a deep breath and follow the sacrum into anatomical extension with inhalation and anatomical flexion with exhalation;
3. Restriction of sacral extension indicates flexion ease;
4. Restriction of sacral flexion indicates extension ease.

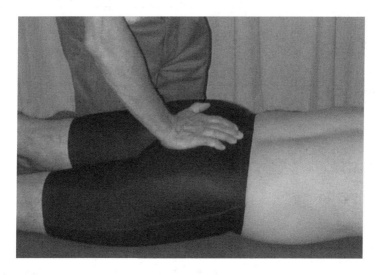

Respiratory motion testing of sacrum

SACRUM SOMATIC DYSFUNCTION DIAGNOSIS

DIAGNOSIS	Seated Flexion Test[1]	Sacral Base Levelness[2]	ILA Levelness	L5 Rotation[3]	Sacral Motion Testing[4]
Left on left torsion[5]	right	anterior right	posterior left	right	extension restriction
Left on right torsion[5]	left	anterior right	posterior left	right	flexion restriction
Right on right torsion[5]	left	anterior left	posterior right	left	extension restriction
Right on left torsion[5]	right	anterior left	posterior right	left	flexion restriction
Left unilateral flexion[6]	left	anterior left	posterior left	–	extension restriction
Left unilateral extension[6]	left	anterior right	posterior right	–	flexion restriction
Right unilateral flexion[6]	right	anterior right	posterior right	–	extension restriction
Right unilateral extension[6]	right	anterior left	posterior left	–	flexion restriction

[1] With a sacral torsion the seated flexion test is positive on the opposite side of the involved oblique axis.

[2] With a sacral torsion the sacrum is rotated to the opposite side of the anterior sacral base.

[3] With a sacral torsion L5 is rotated to the opposite side of sacral rotation. If L5 is rotated to the same side as the sacrum the dysfunction is termed a sacral rotation.

[4] Motion testing can be done with the lumbosacral spring test, backward bending test, respiratory motion testing, or axis motion testing.

[5] Torsions are named for the direction on the axis: Left on left torsion = rotation left on a left oblique axis.

[6] Also known as sacral shear.

KEY TO FIGURE[1]: Findings for a left on left sacral torsion

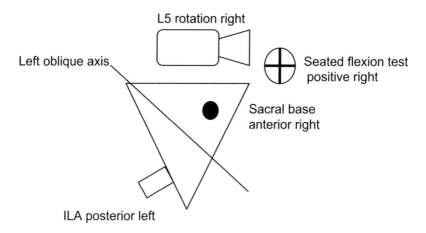

L5 rotation right

Left oblique axis

Seated flexion test positive right

Sacral base anterior right

ILA posterior left

[1] Figure adapted with permission from Graham KE. *Outline of Muscle-Energy Techniques*. Oklahoma College of Osteopathic Medicine and Surgery, Tulsa, 1985.

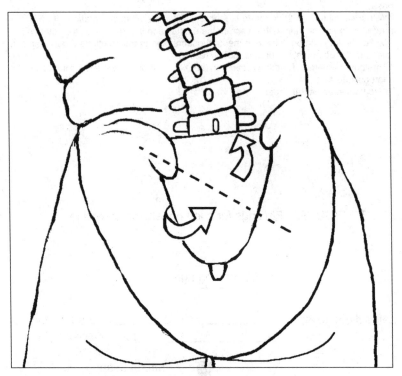

Sacrum rotation left on a left oblique axis

(Drawing by William A. Kuchera, DO, FAAO)

SACRUM COUNTERSTRAIN

Indication: Sacrum tender point associated with back pain, pelvic pain, and other problems.

Relative contraindications: Acute sacral fracture.

Technique (prone):

1. Locate the tender point on the posterior surface of the sacrum, labeling it 10/10;
2. Use your palm to push firmly into the sacrum as far from the tender point as possible, avoiding pressure on the coccyx;
3. Retest for tenderness;
4. Fine tune this position with slightly more or less sacral pressure until tenderness is 2/10 or less;
5. Hold the position of relief for 90 seconds while keeping a finger on the tender point;
6. Slowly remove sacral pressure and retest for tenderness.

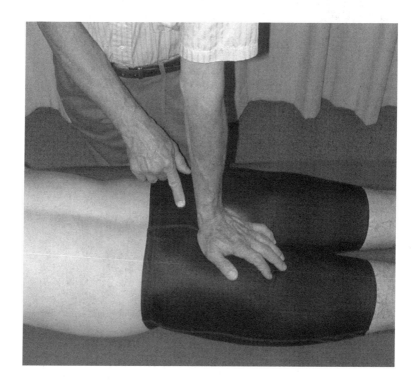

Sacrum tender point and treatment position

MID-POLE SACROILIAC COUNTERSTRAIN

Indication: Mid-pole sacroiliac tender point associated with back pain, pelvic pain, hip pain, and other problems.

Relative contraindications: Severe hip arthritis, deep venous thrombosis in involved leg.

Technique (prone):

1. Locate the tender point by pushing medially onto the lateral sacral margin inferior to the PSIS, labeling it 10/10;
2. Bend the knee on the tender point side and slightly abduct, flex, and externally rotate the hip until tenderness is 2/10 or less;
3. Hold this position for 90 seconds while keeping a finger on the tender point;
4. Slowly return the leg to the table and retest for tenderness.

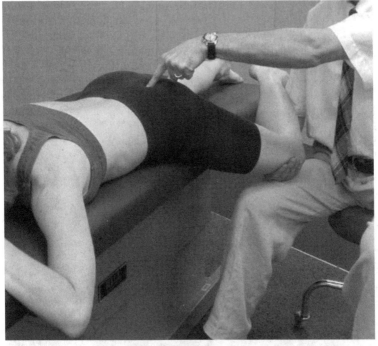

Mid-pole sacroiliac counterstrain

PIRIFORMIS COUNTERSTRAIN

Indication: Piriformis tender point associated with back pain, pelvic pain, hip pain, sciatic neuritis, and other problems.

Relative contraindications: Severe hip arthritis, deep venous thrombosis in involved leg.

Technique (prone):

1. Locate the tender point in the mid-buttock halfway between the top of the greater trochanter and the mid-line of the sacrum, labeling it 10/10;
2. Bend the knee on the tender point side, flex the hip 90°, and abduct and externally rotate the hip until tenderness is 2/10 or less;
3. Hold this position for 90 seconds while keeping a finger on the tender point;
4. Slowly return the leg to the table and retest for tenderness.

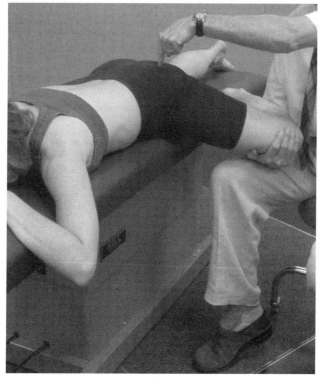

Piriformis counterstrain

SACRAL ROCKING/MYOFASCIAL RELEASE

Indication: Sacral restriction associated with back pain, pelvic pain, sciatic neuritis, constipation, diarrhea, dysmenorrhea, and other problems.

Relative contraindications: Sacral fracture, sacroiliitis, premature labor, placenta previa, placental abruption, bowel obstruction.

Technique (prone, lateral):

1. Place your hands on the sacrum with the bottom hand pointing cephalad and your top hand pointing caudad;
2. Ask the patient to take a deep breath and encourage sacral extension during inhalation by pushing the sacral apex anteriorly;
3. During exhalation encourage sacral flexion by pushing the sacral base anteriorly;
4. Repeat 3-5 times;
5. Alternative technique using myofascial release:
   a) Evaluate flexion by moving the sacral fascia superiorly and extension by moving the sacral fascia inferiorly to determine directions of restriction and laxity;
   b) Indirect: Hold the sacral fascia in the position of laxity and follow any tissue release until completed;
   c) Direct: Hold the sacral fascia in the direction of restriction and apply steady force until tissue give is completed;
6. Retest sacral motion.

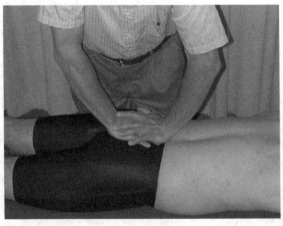

Sacral rocking

SACROILIAC PERCUSSION VIBRATOR

Indications: Restricted sacrum or pelvis motion associated with back pain, pelvic pain, or other problems.

Relative contraindications: Acute fracture, sacroiliitis, undiagnosed radiculopathy, intrapelvic cancer, hip replacement, pregnancy.

Technique (lateral):

1. With the patient lying on the non-restricted side with knees and hips flexed, place your monitoring hand over the greater trochanter and place the vibrating percussor pad lightly on the sacral base;
2. Adjust pad speed, pressure, and angle until vibrations are palpated as strong by the monitoring hand, avoiding pad bouncing;
3. Maintain contact until the force and rhythm of vibration returns to that of normal tissue;
4. Alternative technique:
   a) Allow the monitoring hand to be pulled toward the pad, resisting any other direction of hand pull;
   b) Maintain percussion until the monitoring hand is pushed away from the pad;
5. Slowly release the monitoring hand and the percussion vibrator and retest motion.

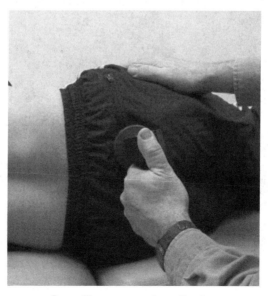

Sacroiliac percussion vibrator

SACRUM FACILITATED OSCILLATORY RELEASE

Indication: Sacral somatic dysfunction associated with back pain, pelvic pain, or other problems.

Relative contraindications: Acute fracture, significant patient guarding.

Technique (prone):

1. Place the heel of your cephalad hand on the lumbar or thoracic transverse processes and the heel of your other hand on the posterior prominence of the sacrum;
2. Localize as appropriate using your radial or ulnar styloid process to make contact with a particular segment;
3. Initiate oscillatory motion of the trunk by rhythmically moving the cephalad hand right and left;
4. Direct your corrective force through the caudad hand against the most posterior portion of the sacrum;
5. Continue vertebral oscillation or modify its force until sacrum mobility improves.

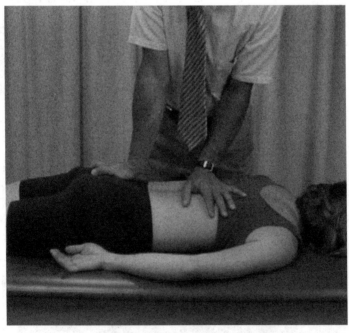

Sacrum facilitated oscillatory release

FORWARD SACRAL TORSION MUSCLE ENERGY

Indication: Forward sacral torsion or rotation (left on left, right on right) associated with back pain, pelvic pain, hip pain, and other problems.

Relative contraindications: Acute sacroiliac sprain, acute sacrum fracture, severe knee arthritis, deep venous thrombosis, premature labor.

Technique (lateral Sims):

1. Sit or stand beside the patient who is lying on the axis side with the chest down on the table;
2. Flex the knees and hips until motion is felt at the lumbosacral junction, usually at least 90° hip flexion;
3. Allow the legs to hang down off the table with thighs supported by your leg or a pillow to avoid pressure from the table;
4. Monitor the anterior sacral base and ask the patient to push the feet toward the ceiling for 3-5 seconds against your equal resistance;
5. Slowly move the legs toward the floor to a new restrictive barrier;
6. Repeat 3-5 times or until return of sacral mobility;
7. Retest sacroiliac motion or sacral symmetry.

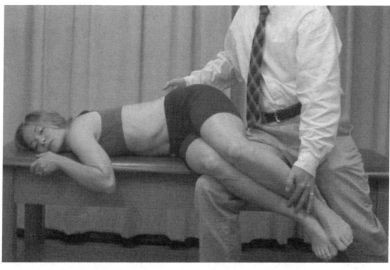

Muscle energy for right on right sacral torsion

BACKWARD SACRAL TORSION MUSCLE ENERGY

Indication: Backward sacral torsion or rotation (left on right, right on left) associated with back pain, pelvic pain, hip pain, and other problems.

Relative contraindications: Acute sacroiliac sprain, acute sacrum fracture, severe hip arthritis, deep venous thrombosis, premature labor.

Technique (lateral recumbent):

1. Sit or stand in front of the patient who is lying on the axis side with the upper back on the table;
2. Extend the leg on the table until motion is felt at the lumbosacral junction;
3. Flex the top leg and place the foot behind the other knee;
4. Hold the shoulder to prevent the patient from rolling and allow the flexed knee to hang down off the table;
5. Ask the patient to push the flexed knee toward the ceiling for 3-5 seconds against your equal resistance;
6. Slowly move the knee toward the floor to a new restrictive barrier;
7. Repeat 3-5 times or until sacral mobility returns;
8. Retest sacroiliac motion or sacral symmetry.

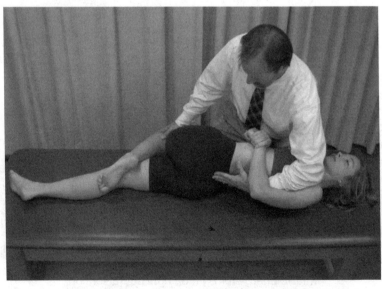

Muscle energy for left on right sacral torsion

SACRAL EXTENSION MUSCLE ENERGY

Indication: Unilateral or bilateral sacral extension associated with back pain, pelvis pain, hip pain, and other problems.

Relative contraindications: Acute sacroiliac sprain, acute sacrum fracture, premature labor.

Technique (prone):

1. Stand facing the patient's feet on the side of the unilateral extension;
2. Place your thenar or hypothenar eminence on the involved sacral base and push it anteriorly and inferiorly by leaning into it. For a bilateral sacral extension push on both sides of the sacral base;
3. Use your other hand to slightly abduct and internally rotate the lower extremity on the involved side;
4. While the patient takes a deep breath, resist sacral extension during inhalation and push the sacrum into flexion during exhalation;
5. Repeat 3-5 times or until sacral mobility returns;
6. Retest sacroiliac motion or sacral symmetry.

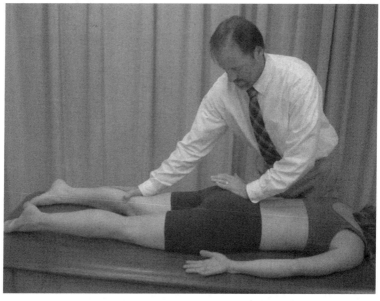

Muscle energy for left unilateral extension

SACRAL FLEXION MUSCLE ENERGY

Indication: Unilateral or bilateral sacral flexion associated with back pain, pelvis pain, hip pain, and other problems.

Relative contraindications: Acute sacroiliac sprain, sacroiliac joint hypermobility, acute sacrum fracture, premature labor.

Technique (prone):

1. Stand facing the patient's head on the side of the unilateral flexion;
2. Place your thenar or hypothenar eminence on the involved inferior lateral angle and push it anteriorly and superiorly by leaning into it. For a bilateral sacral flexion push on both ILAs;
3. Use your other hand to slightly abduct and internally rotate the lower extremity on the involved side;
4. While the patient takes a deep breath, push the sacrum into extension during inhalation and resist sacral flexion during exhalation;
5. Repeat 3-5 times or until sacral mobility returns;
6. Retest sacroiliac motion or sacral symmetry.

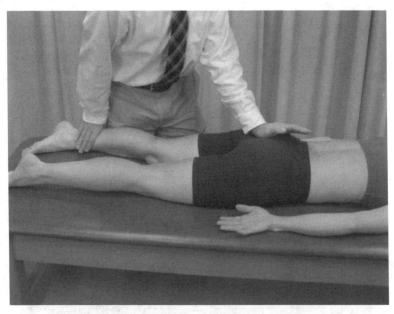

Muscle energy for left unilateral flexion

UNILATERAL SACRAL FLEXION THRUST

Indication: Unilateral sacral flexion (sacral shear) associated with back pain, pelvis pain, hip pain, and other problems.

Relative contraindications: Acute sacroiliac sprain, acute sacrum fracture, hip or knee instability, premature labor.

Technique (supine or lateral):

1. Stabilize the inferior lateral angle (ILA) on the side of the unilateral flexion by placing a wedge on its inferior surface (supine one person technique) or by having an assistant push the ILA superiorly and anteriorly (lateral two person technique);
2. Standing at the foot of the table, grasp the ankle above the malleoli with both hands and slightly abduct and internally rotate the leg on the unilateral flexion side;
3. Ask the patient to take a deep breath and during exhalation apply a firm and quick tug down the leg;
4. Retest sacroiliac motion or sacral symmetry.

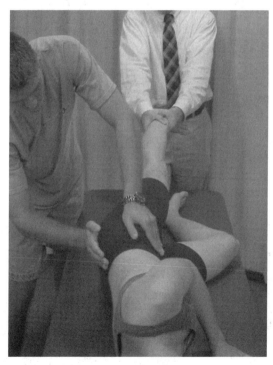

Two person thrust for left unilateral flexion

PIRIFORMIS POSITION OF EASE

1. Lie on your back with legs propped up on a chair or stool;
2. Cross your ankles with the foot on the side of back pain on top;
3. Let your knees fall apart;
4. If comfortable, take a few deep breaths and rest in this position for 2-5 minutes;
5. Slowly uncross your legs, bring them down, and roll to one side before getting up;
6. Use this position 2-4 times a day or as needed for pain relief.

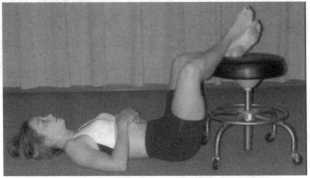

Piriformis position of ease

PIRIFORMIS STRETCH

1. Lie on your back and place one foot on top of the other knee;
2. Grasp the outside of the bent knee with your opposite hand;
3. Allow your bent leg to slowly fall over the other leg as far as it will comfortably go;
4. Pull the bent knee down toward the floor with the opposite hand;
5. Take a few deep breaths and stretch for 10-20 seconds;
6. Repeat to the opposite side;
7. Do this stretch 1-4 times a day.

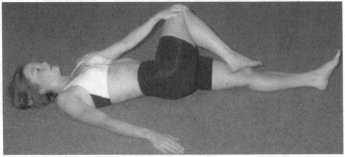

Piriformis stretch

SACROILIAC MOBILIZATION

1. Lie on your back and bend one leg up, grasping the knee with both hands. If the knee hurts, instead grasp the thigh behind the knee;
2. Pull the knee up toward your opposite shoulder as far as it will comfortably go;
3. Take a few deep breaths and with each exhalation pull the knee a little farther toward the opposite shoulder;
4. Use the opposite hand to pull the knee across your abdomen as you extend the leg;
5. Repeat for the other side;
6. Do up to twice a day if helpful.

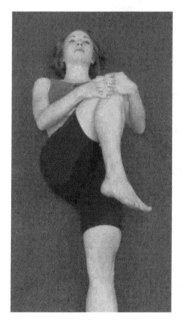
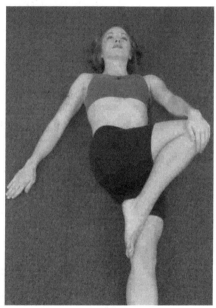

Flexion stretch   Adduction with extension

SACROILIAC SIDEBENDING MOBILIZATION

1. Lie on your back with knees bent and feet flat on the floor;
2. Reach your left hip outward and up toward your left shoulder as far as it will go;
3. Reach your right hip outward and up toward your right shoulder as far as it will go;
4. Repeat 1-3 times;
5. Do up to twice a day if helpful.

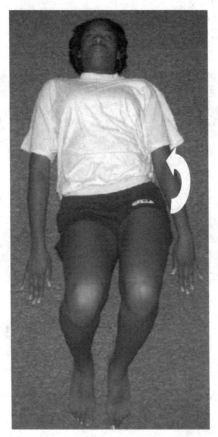

Sacroiliac sidebending mobilization

SACRAL NOTES (cont.)

LUMBAR NOTES

Diagnosis of Lumbar Somatic Dysfunction

1. Screening tests
   Hip drop test – p.124
   Lumbosacral fascial rotation – p.124
2. Palpation
   a) Lumbar tender points – pp.125-126
   b) Lumbar tension – p.127
3. Lumbar rotation testing – p.128
4. Lumbar somatic dysfunction – p.129
5. Neurological exam before treatment of low back problems:
   a) Deep tendon reflexes
       Patella reflex – L4 nerve root
       Achilles reflex – S1 nerve root
   b) Muscle strength
       Foot inversion – L4 nerve root
       Great toe dorsiflexion – L5 nerve root
       Foot eversion – S1 nerve root
   c) Sensation testing
   d) Straight leg raising test for low back and leg pain or paresthesias

Treatment of Lumbar Somatic Dysfunction

1. OMT
   Thoracolumbar kneading/stretching – p.130
   T10-L5 posterior counterstrain – p.131
   Lower pole L5 counterstrain – p.132
   T9-L5 anterior counterstrain – p.133
   Lumbosacral myofascial release – see p.79
   Lumbosacral compression/decompression – p.134
   Lumbar soft tissue facilitated positional release – p.135
   Lumbar flexion facilitated positional release – p.136
   Lumbar extension facilitated positional release – p.137
   Lumbar percussion vibrator – p.138
   Thoracolumbar facilitated oscillatory release – p.139
   Lumbar muscle energy, lateral – p.140
   Lumbar muscle energy, lateral recumbent – p.141
   Lumbar muscle energy/thrust, seated – p.142
   Lumbar articulatory, seated – p.143
   Lumbosacral articulatory/thrust, supine – p.144
   Lumbar thrust, lateral recumbent – p.145
2. Exercises
   Lumbar position of ease – p.146
   Lumbar extensor stretch – p.146
   Lumbar mobilization – p.147
   Thoracolumbar stretch/mobilization – p.147
3. Thermal therapy
   Heat 20-30 minutes 4-6 times a day for tension or stiffness
   Cold 15-20 minutes 4-6 times a day for pain relief
4. Stabilization
   Lumbosacral support belt for overuse strain
   Prolotherapy for ligament laxity and joint hypermobility

HIP DROP TEST

1. Ask the standing patient to bend one knee and drop that hip which induces lumbar sidebending away from the dropped hip;
2. Observe lumbar sidebending and amount of hip drop which is normally $\geq 25°$;
3. Hip drop $< 25°$ (positive test) indicates restricted lumbar sidebending toward the opposite side of the dropped hip.

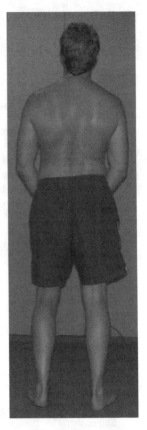

Left hip drop test
(sidebending right)

LUMBOSACRAL FASCIAL ROTATION

1. With the patient supine, place your palms over the skin of the lateral pelvis and simultaneously lift one side while pushing the other side posteriorly to induce lumbosacral fascia rotation;
2. Repeat for the other direction to identify rotational restriction and laxity.

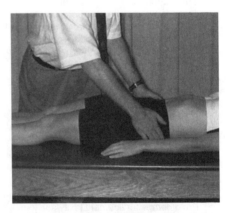

Lumbosacral fascial rotation

LUMBAR TENDER POINTS

1. Palpate for posterior lumbar tender points at the following locations:

   a) **Posterior T10-L5** – spinous processes or 1/2-1" lateral;
   b) **Posterior L3** – gluteal musculature halfway between posterior L4 and L5;
   c) **Posterior L4** – iliac crest in posterior axillary line;
   d) **Posterior L5** (upper pole L5) – superior surface of posterior superior iliac spine (PSIS) at insertion of iliolumbar ligament;
   e) **Lower pole L5** – inferior surface of the PSIS.

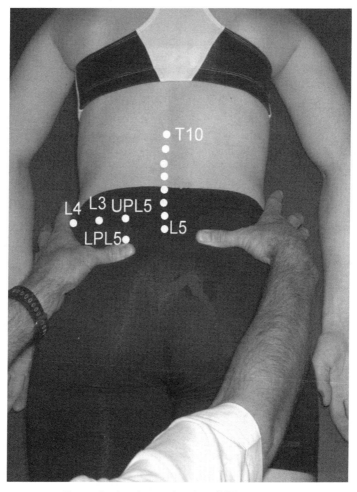

Posterior lumbar palpation (LPL5 shown)

2. Palpate for anterior lumbar tender points at the following locations:

a) **Anterior T9** – 1/2-1" superior to umbilicus;
b) **Anterior T10** – 1" below umbilicus;
c) **Anterior T11** – 2" below umbilicus;
d) **Anterior T12** – inner aspect of iliac crest in mid-axillary line;
e) **Anterior L1** – 1/2" medial to anterior superior iliac spine (ASIS);
f) **Anterior L2** – medial surface of anterior inferior iliac spine (AIIS);
g) **Anterior L3** – lateral surface of AIIS;
h) **Anterior L4** – inferior surface of AIIS;
i) **Anterior L5** – pubic ramus 1/2" lateral to pubic symphysis.

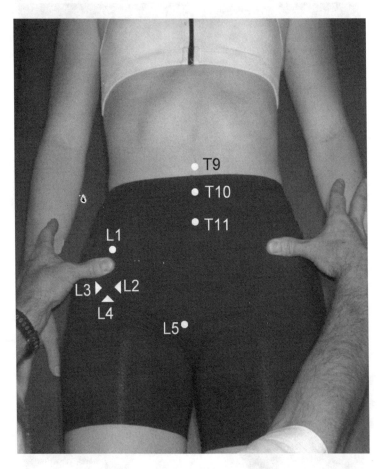

Anterior lumbar tender points
(ASIS palpation shown, AT12 not shown)

126

LUMBAR TENSION PALPATION

1. With the patient seated or prone, palpate the lumbar paraspinal area, comparing right and left sides for increased fullness;
2. Fullness may be due to muscle tension, edema, or vertebral rotation to that side;
3. Vertebral rotation multiple segments = neutral or type 1 somatic dysfunction with sidebending to opposite side;
4. Vertebral rotation single segment = non-neutral or type 2 somatic dysfunction with sidebending to same side – test flexion and extension;
5. Rotation worse in flexion = extension somatic dysfunction; Rotation worse in extension = flexion somatic dysfunction.

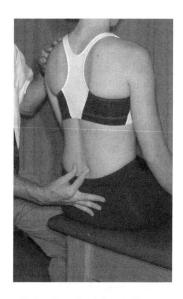

Palpation for L3 rotation

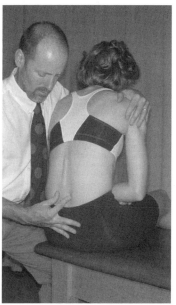

Flexion testing

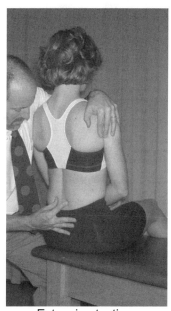

Extension testing

LUMBAR ROTATION TESTING

1. With the patient prone or seated, place your thumbs on a lumbar vertebra's transverse processes located an inch lateral to the spinous process;
2. Push anteriorly on the right transverse process to induce rotation left;
    Push anteriorly on the left transverse process to induce rotation right;
3. Restricted rotation left = rotated right;
    Restricted rotation right = rotation left.

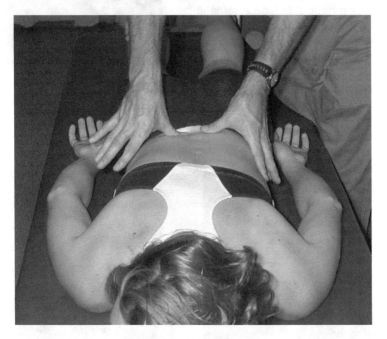

Testing L4 rotation left

Findings	NEUTRAL OR TYPE 1	NON-NEUTRAL OR TYPE 2
Paraspinal fullness (rotation)	Multiple vertebrae	One vertebra
Sidebending	Opposite rotation	Same as rotation
Flexion or extension result	Minimal change	Fullness increases
Somatic dysfunction	N Rx Sy	F or E Rx Sx
Visceral association	Rare	Possible

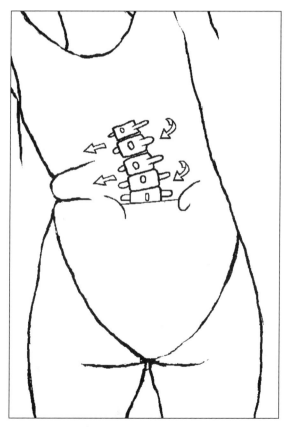

Neutral, sidebending left, rotation right

(Drawing by William A. Kuchera, DO, FAAO)

129

THORACOLUMBAR KNEADING/STRETCHING

Indications: Thoracic or lumbar paraspinal muscle tension associated with back pain, chest wall pain, and other problems.

Relative contraindications: Acute lumbar strain and sprain, acute vertebral or rib fracture.

Technique (prone):

1. Stand on the opposite side and place your cephalad palm on the tense muscle lateral to the spinous processes;
2. Grasp the ASIS on the side of tension with your caudad hand;
3. Slowly knead the tension by leaning into your cephalad hand with the arm straightened to push the muscle anteriorly and laterally, avoiding sliding over the skin;
4. Simultaneously stretch the tense muscle by slowly pulling your caudad hand posteriorly to lift the ASIS until resistance is felt;
5. Repeat simultaneous kneading and stretching until tension is reduced.

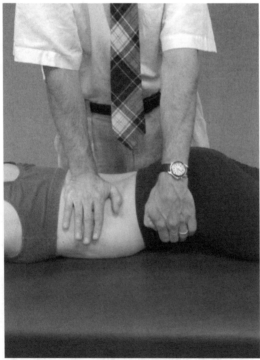

Thoracolumbar kneading/stretching

T10-L5 POSTERIOR COUNTERSTRAIN

Indication: Posterior T10-L5 tender point associated with back pain, pelvis pain, chest pain, and other problems.

Relative contraindications: Acute fracture, hip dislocation, severe hip osteoarthritis.

Technique (prone):

1. Locate the tender point, labeling it 10/10;
2. Stand on the opposite side and lift the thigh on the side of the tender point to extend the hip;
3. Retest for tenderness;
4. Fine tune this position with slightly more hip extension, abduction, or adduction until tenderness is 2/10 or less;
5. Hold the position of relief for 90 seconds while keeping a finger on the tender point;
6. Slowly and passively return the hip to neutral and retest for tenderness.

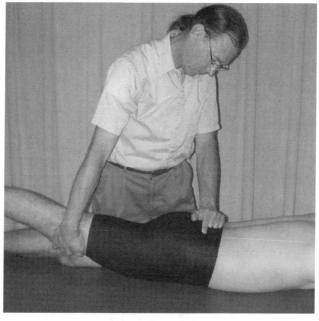

L3 posterior tender point and treatment position

LOWER POLE L5 COUNTERSTRAIN

Indication: Lower pole L5 tender point associated with back pain, pelvic pain, hip pain, and other problems.

Relative contraindications: Acute fracture, hip dislocation, severe hip osteoarthritis.

Technique (prone):

1. Locate the tender point on the inferior aspect of the posterior superior iliac spine, labeling it 10/10;
2. Flex the hip and knee 90° and retest for tenderness;
3. Fine tune this position with slight hip adduction until tenderness is 2/10 or less;
4. Hold the position of relief for 90 seconds while keeping a finger on the tender point;
5. Slowly and passively return the leg to the table and retest for tenderness.

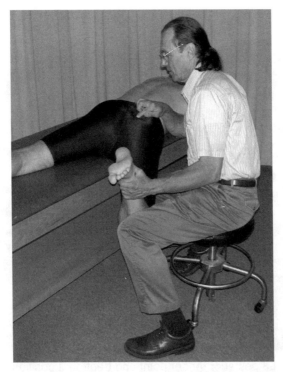

Lower pole L5 tender point and treatment position

Indication: Anterior T9-L5 tender point associated with back pain, pelvic pain, chest wall pain, abdominal pain, and other problems.

Relative contraindications: Acute lumbar fracture, acute lumbar strain and sprain.

Technique (supine):

1. Stand beside the patient and locate the tender point, labeling it 10/10;
2. Passively flex the knees and hips 90° and retest for tenderness;
3. Fine tune this position with increased hip flexion and slight rotation or sidebending of the knees until tenderness is 2/10 or less;
4. Hold the position of relief for 90 seconds while keeping a finger on the tender point;
5. Slowly and passively return the legs to the table and retest for tenderness.

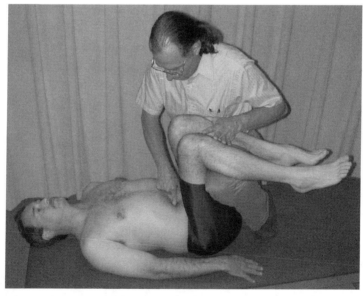

Anterior T10 tender point and treatment position

LUMBOSACRAL COMPRESSION/DECOMPRESSION

Indication: Lumbosacral tension related to back pain, sacroiliac pain, pelvic pain, and other problems.

Relative contraindications: Acute lumbar or sacral fracture.

Technique (prone or lateral):

1. Place one hand on the sacrum pointing caudad and the other hand on the lumbar spine pointing cephalad. Hands may also be pointed in the same direction;
2. Slowly pull your palms together to compress the lumbosacral fascia and then push your palms apart to decompress the lumbosacral fascia, determining directions of laxity and restriction;
3. Indirect: Move the lumbosacral fascia to its position of laxity and follow any tissue release until completed;
4. Direct: Move the lumbosacral fascia into its restriction and apply steady force until tissue give is completed;
5. Retest lumbosacral compression and decompression.

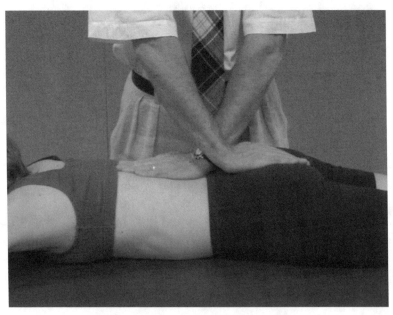

Lumbosacral compression/decompression

LUMBAR SOFT TISSUE FACILITATED POSITIONAL RELEASE[1]

Indications: Lumbar paraspinal tension associated with back pain, pelvic pain, hip pain, and other problems.

Relative contraindications: Acute lumbar fracture, severe hip arthritis.

Technique (prone):

1. Place a pillow under the abdomen to decrease lumbar lordosis;
2. Stand on the side of paraspinal tension, palpate the tension with your cephalad hand, and grasp the outside of the opposite distal thigh with your other hand;
3. Extend and adduct the leg until tension is reduced;
4. Hold this position for 3–5 seconds until tension release is completed;
5. Slowly lower the leg to the table and retest for tension.

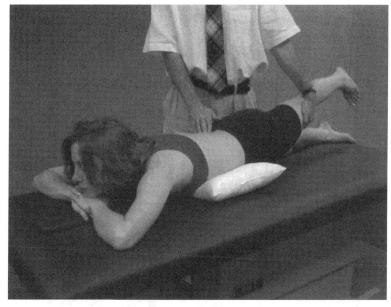

Lumbar soft tissue facilitated positional release

LUMBAR FLEXION FACILITATED POSITIONAL RELEASE[1]

Indications: Lumbar flexion somatic dysfunction associated with back pain and other problems.

Relative contraindications: Severe hip arthritis.

Technique (prone):

1. Place a pillow under the abdomen to decrease lumbar lordosis;
2. Sit on the side of lumbar rotation and palpate the paraspinal tension;
3. Flex the hip on the side of lumbar rotation by dropping the knee off the table until paraspinal tension decreases;
4. Add compression by lifting the knee or traction by letting the knee drop to further reduce paraspinal tension;
5. Hold this position for 3–5 seconds until tension release is completed and slowly return the leg to the table;
6. Remove the pillow and retest lumbar rotation.

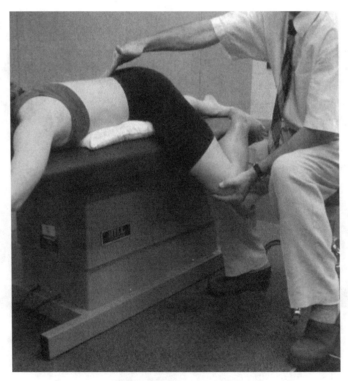

FPR for L5 FRS left

LUMBAR EXTENSION FACILITATED POSITIONAL RELEASE[1]

Indications: Lumbar extension somatic dysfunction associated with back pain and other problems.

Relative contraindications: Severe hip arthritis.

Technique (prone):

1. Position the patient with the hip on the side of lumbar rotation close to the edge of the table;
2. Place a pillow under the abdomen to decrease lumbar lordosis and another pillow between the mid-thigh and table;
3. Sit on the side of lumbar rotation and palpate the paraspinal tension;
4. Abduct the leg to create lumbar side bending to the side of lumbar rotation;
5. Hold the ankle and internally rotate the lower leg until motion is felt at the dysfunctional segment;
6. Push the leg downward to flex the hip until motion is felt at the dysfunctional segment;
7. Hold this position for 3–5 seconds until tension release is completed and slowly return the leg to the table;
8. Remove the pillows and retest lumbar rotation.

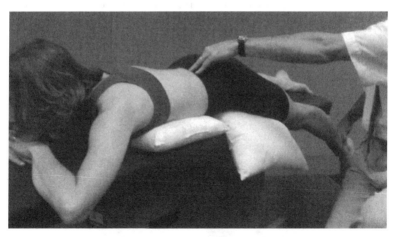

FPR for L5 ERS left

LUMBAR PERCUSSION VIBRATOR

Indications: Lumbar somatic dysfunction associated with back pain and other problems.

Relative contraindications: Acute fracture, undiagnosed radiculopathy, lumbar or intrapelvic cancer, hip replacement, pregnancy.

Technique (lateral):

1. With the patient lying on the non-restricted side with knees and hips flexed, place your monitoring hand over the greater trochanter;
2. Place the vibrating percussion pad lightly on the involved lumbar spinous processes perpendicular to the surface avoiding pad bouncing;
3. Alter pad speed, pressure, and angle until vibrations are palpated as strong by the monitoring hand;
4. Maintain contact until the force and rhythm of vibration returns to that of normal tissue;
5. Alternative technique:
   a) Allow the monitoring hand to be pulled toward the pad, resisting any other direction of hand pull;
   b) Maintain percussion until the monitoring hand is pushed away from the pad;
6. Slowly release the monitoring hand and the percussion vibrator and retest tissue texture or motion.

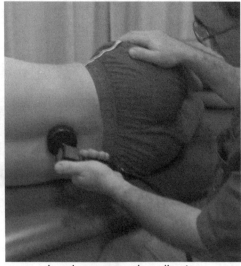

Lumbar percussion vibrator

THORACOLUMBAR FACILITATED OSCILLATORY RELEASE

Indication: Lumbar or thoracic somatic dysfunction associated with back pain, chest wall pain, or other problems.

Relative contraindications: Acute fracture, significant patient guarding.

Technique (prone):

1. Place one hand on the sacrum and the heel of your other hand over the posterior transverse processes or ribs;
2. Localize as appropriate using your radial or ulnar styloid process to make contact with a particular segment;
3. Initiate oscillatory motion of the pelvis by rhythmically moving your sacral hand right and left;
4. Add corrective force through your cephalad hand onto the transverse processes or ribs;
5. Continue pelvic oscillation or modify its force until you feel tension is reduced or mobility improves.

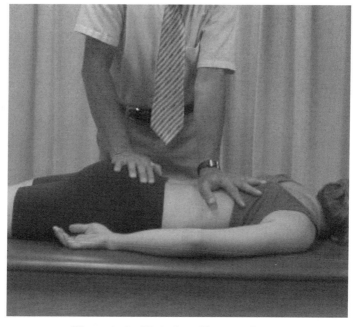

Thoracic facilitated oscillatory release

LUMBAR MUSCLE ENERGY – LATERAL

Indication: Restricted multi-segment lumbar rotation associated with back pain, scoliosis, and other problems.

Relative contraindications: Acute lumbar sprain, undiagnosed radiculopathy, acute vertebral fracture, vertebral cancer or infection.

Technique:

1. Stand in front of the patient who is lying with the vertebral rotation side up;
2. Flex the hips until you feel motion in the middle of the restricted segments;
3. Lift both ankles until you feel sidebending in the middle of the restricted segments;
4. Ask the patient to push the ankles down toward the table for 3-5 seconds against your equal resistance;
5. Slowly lift the ankles to a new lumbar sidebending restrictive barrier;
6. Repeat 3-5 times or until lumbar mobility returns;
7. Retest lumbar rotation.

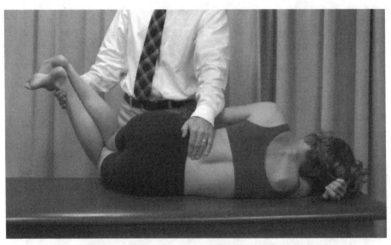

Muscle energy for L1-5 N R left S right

LUMBAR MUSCLE ENERGY – LATERAL RECUMBENT

Indication: Restricted lumbar rotation associated with back pain, scoliosis, and other problems.

Relative contraindications: Acute lumbar sprain, undiagnosed radiculopathy, acute vertebral fracture, vertebral cancer or infection.

Technique:

1. Stand in front of the patient who is lying with the side of lumbar rotation toward the table;
2. Flex the upward hip until you feel motion at the restricted segment and tuck the foot behind the other knee;
3. Rotate the back toward the table by pushing the upward shoulder posteriorly and lifting the table-side arm and shoulder until you feel rotation at the restricted segment;
4. Place your forearm across the buttock, lean over top of that arm, and use your other arm to stabilize the patient's shoulder, taking care not to push into the ribs or breast;
5. Ask the patient to push the pelvis backward for 3-5 seconds against your equal resistance;
6. Slowly move the pelvis anteromedially to a new lumbar rotation restrictive barrier;
7. Repeat 3-5 times or until lumbar mobility returns;
8. Retest lumbar rotation.

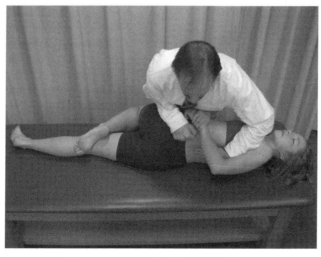

Muscle energy for L3 rotated right

Indication: Restricted lumbar or thoracic rotation associated with back pain, scoliosis, and other problems.

Relative contraindications: Acute lumbar sprain, joint hypermobility, undiagnosed radiculopathy, acute vertebral fracture, vertebral cancer or infection.

Technique:

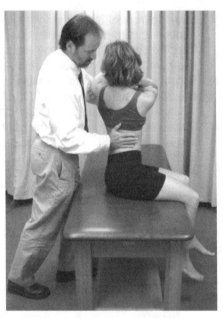

ME for L1-5 N R right S left

1. Standing behind the seated patient, place your thenar eminence on the posterior transverse process(es);
2. Reach across the upper chest with your other hand and arm to control the patient's shoulders and trunk;
3. Move the trunk into the rotation, sidebending, and flexion-extension restrictive barriers until you feel movement at the restricted segment(s);
4. Ask the patient to straighten the trunk and/or shoulders for 3-5 seconds against your equal resistance;
5. Slowly move the trunk to new restrictive barriers as you push anterior into the posterior transverse process(es);
6. Repeat 3-5 times or until lumbar mobility returns;
7. Add a thrust if needed by a short and quick anterior push into the posterior transverse process(es) as you simultaneously move the trunk into its restrictive barriers;
8. Retest lumbar rotation.

Indications: Restricted lumbar rotation associated with back pain, pelvic pain, and other problems.

Relative contraindications: Joint inflammation, joint hypermobility, acute sprain, acute fracture, vertebral cancer, undiagnosed lumbosacral radiculopathy.

Technique:

1. Sit behind the seated patient and place your thumb on the inferior facet of the restricted vertebral segment to stabilize it;
2. Place your other hand on the shoulder and slowly induce trunk movement into the rotation, sidebending, and flexion-extension positions of ease;
   a) Locked closed facet: Induce extension and sidebending-rotation toward it;
   b) Locked open facet: Induce flexion and sidebending-rotation away from it;
3. Slowly move the torso into the restrictive barrier for all planes and then slowly return to the positions of ease;
4. Repeat if necessary, adding an isometric contraction and release by having the patient take a deep breath or push against your counterforce in any plane;
5. Retest lumbar rotation.

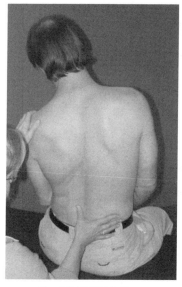

2a: L2 E RS left
(locked closed left)

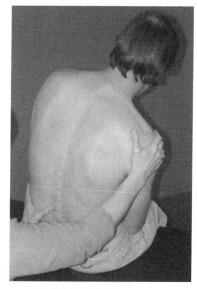

2b: L2 F RS right
(locked open left)

LUMBOSACRAL ARTICULATORY/THRUST – SUPINE

Indications: Restricted lumbar rotation or sacroiliac joint mobility associated with back pain, pelvic pain, and other problems.

Relative contraindications: Joint inflammation, joint hypermobility, acute sprain, acute fracture, vertebral cancer, undiagnosed lumbosacral radiculopathy.

Technique (supine):

1. Ask the patient to interlock his or her fingers behind the head;
2. Stand to one side of the patient, use the palm of your caudad hand to hold the opposite anterior superior iliac spine (ASIS), and reach your cephalad hand over and through the patient's opposite elbow, placing the back of your hand on the sternum;
3. Lean into the ASIS and slowly pull the patient's arm toward you until reaching a rotation and flexion restrictive barrier;
4. If needed, apply a short and quick thrust posteriorly into the ASIS;
5. Retest lumbar rotation or sacroiliac mobility.

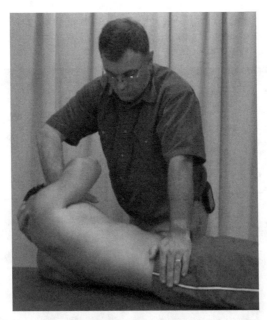

Lumbosacral articulatory/thrust (OB roll)

Indication: Restricted lumbar rotation associated with back pain, scoliosis, and other problems.

Relative contraindications: Acute lumbar sprain, lumbar joint hypermobility, undiagnosed radiculopathy, acute vertebral fracture, acute herniated or ruptured disc, vertebral cancer or infection.

Technique:

1. Stand in front of the patient who is lying on the side of lumbar rotation;
2. Flex the upward hip until you feel motion at the restricted segment and then tuck the foot behind the other knee;
3. Rotate the back toward the table by lifting the table-side arm until you feel rotation at the restricted segment;
4. Use your cephalad arm to stabilize the shoulder, place your other forearm across the buttock, and lean over top of that arm;
5. Ask the patient to take a deep breath and during exhalation slowly push the pelvis anteromedially to take up the rotational slack;
6. At the end of exhalation apply a short quick thrust with your arm and body onto the pelvis in an anteromedial direction;
7. Retest lumbar rotation.

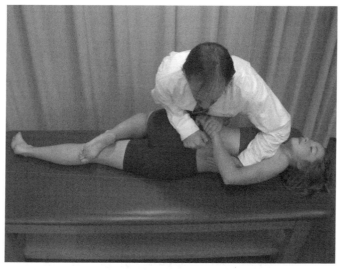

Lateral recumbent thrust for L3 rotated right

LUMBAR POSITION OF EASE

1. Lay face down with a pillow or two under your pelvis on the side of the back pain;
2. If comfortable, take a few deep breaths and rest in this position for 2-5 minutes;
3. Slowly roll to one side before getting up;
4. Use this position 2-4 times a day or as needed for pain relief.

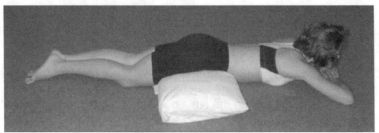
Lumbar position of ease

LUMBAR EXTENSOR STRETCH

1. Lie on your back and grasp both knees with your hands. If knee pain occurs, instead grasp the thighs behind the knees;
2. Use your arms to slowly pull the knees toward the chest as far as they will comfortably go;
3. Take a few deep breaths and stretch for 10-20 seconds;
4. Do this stretch 1-4 times a day.

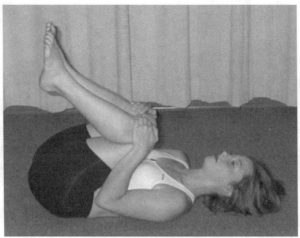
Lumbar extensor stretch

LUMBAR MOBILIZATION[2]

1. Lie on your back with knees bent, feet on the floor, and arms outstretched;
2. Drape one knee over the other and allow the legs to fall to the floor while keeping the shoulders down;
3. Repeat to the other side;
4. Do up to twice a day if helpful.

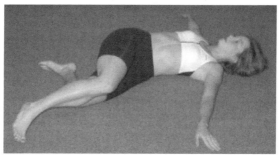

Lumbar mobilization

THORACOLUMBAR STRETCH/MOBILIZATION[2]

1. Sit with your legs straight and hands on the floor behind you;
2. Bend one knee and place the opposite arm against the outside of the bent leg;
3. Slowly turn your trunk toward the bent leg as far as it will comfortably go while pushing the arm into the leg;
4. Take a few deep breaths and stretch for 10-20 seconds;
5. For mobilization, add a short quick push of the arm into the leg to twist the trunk slightly farther;
6. Repeat to the other side;
7. Stretch 1-4 times a day and mobilize up to twice a day.

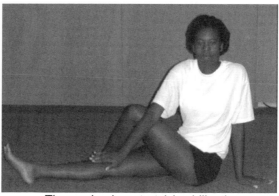

Thoracolumbar stretch/mobilization

REFERENCES

1. Adapted from Schiowitz S, DiGiovanna EL, Dowling DJ. *Chapter 64: Facilitated Positional Release* in Ward RC, Ed. *Foundations for Osteopathic Medicine 2nd Edition.* Lippincott Williams & Wilkins, Philadelphia, 2003.
2. Adapted from Kirk CE. *Biodynamics of self-administered manipulation.* 1977 AAO Yearbook, American Academy of Osteopathy, Colorado Springs, 1979.

THORACIC NOTES

Diagnosis of Thoracic Somatic Dysfunction

Treatment of Thoracic Somatic Dysfunction

1. OMT

2. Exercises

3. Thermal therapy
Heat 20-30 minutes 4-6 times a day for tension or stiffness
Cold 15-20 minutes 4-6 times a day for pain relief

THORACIC TENSION PALPATION

1. With the patient seated or prone, palpate the thoracic paraspinal area, comparing right and left sides for increased fullness;
2. Fullness may be due to muscle tension, edema, or vertebral rotation to that side;
3. Vertebral rotation multiple segments = neutral or type 1 somatic dysfunction with sidebending to the opposite side;
4. Vertebral rotation single segment = non-neutral or type 2 somatic dysfunction with sidebending to the same side: test flexion and extension;

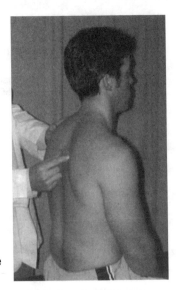

Palpation for T5 rotation

5. Induce passive flexion and extension as follows;
   - T1-6 – flex and extend the head;
   - T7-12 – flex and extend the trunk (see p. 127);
6. Increased tension with flexion = extension somatic dysfunction; Increased tension with extension = flexion somatic dysfunction.

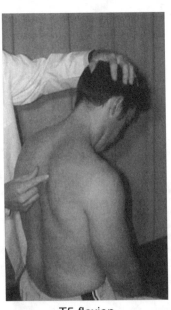

T5 flexion

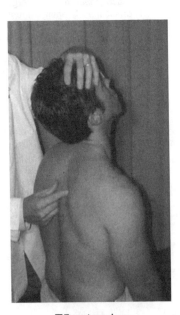

T5 extension

1. Palpate for posterior thoracic tender points at the following locations:

   a) **Posterior T1-T9** – spinous process or 1/2" lateral;
   b) **Posterior T10-T12** – see p. 125.

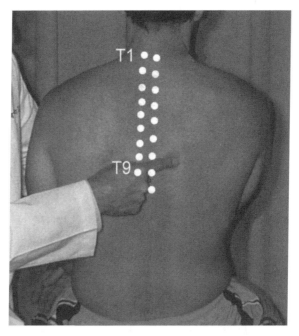

Posterior thoracic tender points
(right T8 shown)

2. Palpate for anterior thoracic tender points at the following locations:

a) **T1** – sternal notch pushing inferiorly;
b) **T2** – middle of manubrium;
c) **T3-T4** – sternum at level of corresponding rib insertion;
d) **T5** – 1" above xiphisternal junction or at rib 5 cartilage;
e) **T6** – xiphisternal junction or at rib 6 cartilage;
f) **T7** – tip of xiphoid process or at rib 7 cartilage;
g) **T8** – 1.5" below xiphoid process or at chondral mass;
h) **T9-T12** – see p. 126.

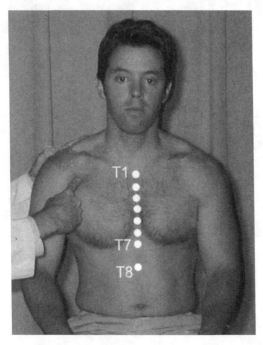

Anterior thoracic tender points
(pectoralis minor palpation shown)

1. With the patient prone, place your thumbs on a thoracic vertebra's transverse processes which are located 1/2-1" lateral to the mid-line as follows (rule of threes):

    T1-3 – transverse processes directly lateral to spinous process;

    T4-6 – transverse processes halfway between spinous process and that of segment above;

    T6-9 – transverse processes directly lateral to spinous process of segment above;

    T10-12 – transverse processes return to directly lateral to spinous process.

2. Push anteriorly on the right transverse process to induce rotation left;

    Push anteriorly on the left transverse process to induce rotation right;

2. Restricted rotation left = rotated right;

    Restricted rotation right = rotation left.

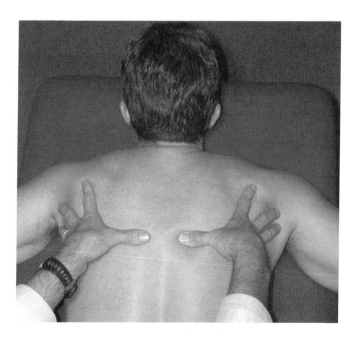

T6 rotation testing

Findings	Neutral or Type 1	Non-Neutral or Type 2
Paraspinal fullness (rotation)	Multiple vertebrae	One vertebra
Sidebending	Opposite rotation	Same as rotation
Flexion or extension result	Minimal change	Fullness increases
Somatic dysfunction	N Rx Sy	F or E Rx Sx
Visceral association	Rare	Possible

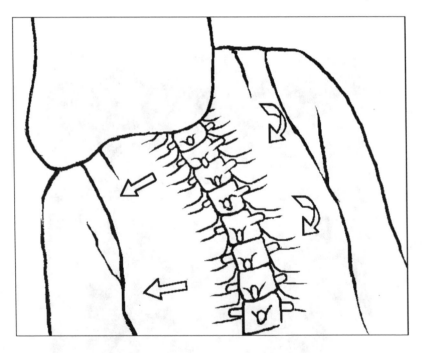

Neutral, sidebending left, rotation right
(Drawing by William A. Kuchera, DO, FAAO)

THORACOLUMBAR KNEADING

Indications: Thoracic or lumbar paraspinal muscle tension associated with back pain, chest wall pain, and other problems.

Relative contraindications: Acute vertebral or rib fracture.

Technique (lateral):

1. Stand facing the patient who is lying on the opposite side of paraspinal muscle tension;
2. Drape the patient's arm over your forearm to move the scapula away from the spine;
3. Grasp the tense muscle with the fingertips of one or both hands;
4. Slowly lean backward to pull the tense muscle laterally, avoiding sliding over the skin;
5. Repeat kneading until tension is reduced.

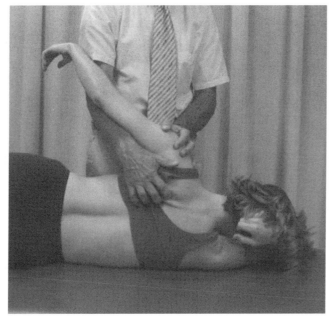

Thoracic kneading

POSTERIOR T1-T9 MIDLINE COUNTERSTRAIN

Indication: Midline posterior T1-T9 tender point associated with back pain, chest pain, neck pain, headache, and other problems.

Relative contraindications: Acute fracture.

Technique (prone):

1. Locate the tender point by pushing anteriorly into the spinous process, labeling it 10/10;
2. Extend the upper thoracic spine by cupping the chin and gently lifting the head;
3. Retest for tenderness;
4. Fine tune this position with slightly more or less extension until tenderness is 2/10 or less;
5. Hold the position of relief for 90 seconds;
6. Slowly and passively return the head to neutral and retest for tenderness.

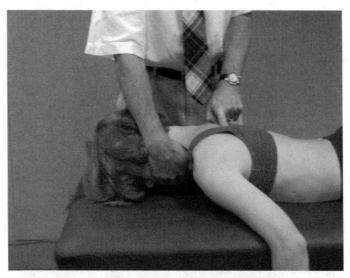

PT5 midline counterstrain

Indication: Lateral posterior T1-T9 tender point associated with back pain, chest pain, shoulder pain, neck pain, headache, and other problems.

Relative contraindications: Acute fracture, shoulder dislocation.

Technique (prone):

1. Locate the tender point lateral to the spinous process, labeling it 10/10;
2. Lift the shoulder on the side of the tender point posteriorly toward the point and retest for tenderness;
3. Fine tune this position with slightly more or less shoulder lift until tenderness is 2/10 or less;
4. Hold the position of relief for 90 seconds;
5. Slowly and passively return the shoulder to neutral and retest for tenderness.

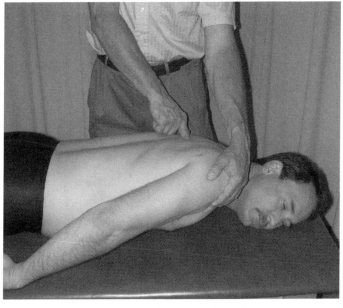

Counterstrain for right lateral PT5

ANTERIOR T1-T8 COUNTERSTRAIN

Indication: Anterior T1-T8 tender point associated with back pain, chest wall pain, and other problems.

Relative contraindications: Acute thoracic or rib fracture, acute cervical fracture, or dislocation.

Technique (supine):

1. Stand at the head of the table and locate the tender point, labeling it 10/10;
2. Flex the neck and upper back until tenderness is reduced, supporting the patient in this position with your arm, thigh, or abdomen;
3. Retest for tenderness and fine tune this position with slightly more or less flexion until tenderness is 2/10 or less;
4. Hold the position of relief for 90 seconds;
5. Slowly and passively return the patient to neutral and retest for tenderness.

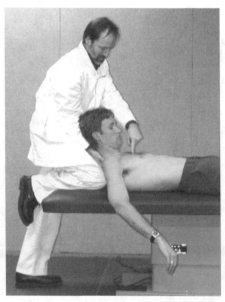

AT4 tender point and treatment position

THORACOLUMBAR MYOFASCIAL RELEASE
(diaphragm, thoracic outlet)

Indication: Restricted thoracolumbar rotation related to back pain, chest wall pain, edema, shortness of breath, and other problems.

Relative contraindications: Acute costochondral subluxation.

Technique (supine or prone):

1. Place one hand across the chondral masses of the lower ribs and your other hand across the thoracolumbar spinous processes. Alternatively, place a hand on either side of the lower rib cage;
2. Indirect: Gently compress your hands together or rotate the fascia under your hands to the position of laxity, maintaining fascial laxity and following any tissue release until completed;
3. Direct: Gently move the thoracolumbar fascia into its superior-inferior, rotation, and sidebending restrictions and apply steady force until tissue give is completed;
4. Retest thoracolumbar rotation.

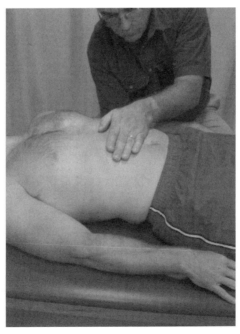

Thoracolumbar myofascial release

CERVICOTHORACIC MYOFASCIAL RELEASE (thoracic inlet)

Indication: Restricted cervicothoracic rotation related to neck pain, headache, back pain, chest wall pain, edema, shortness of breath, and other problems.

Relative contraindications: Acute clavicle fracture.

Technique (supine):

1. Sit at the head of the table and place your hands across the top of the shoulders with fingertips on upper ribs and thumbs overlying the scapulae;
2. Move one hand anteriorly and the other hand posteriorly to induce fascial rotation and repeat for the other direction to identify rotational restriction and laxity;
3. Indirect: Rotate the cervicothoracic fascia to its position of laxity and follow any tissue release until completed;
4. Direct: Rotate the cervicothoracic fascia into its restriction and apply steady force until tissue give is completed;
5. Retest cervicothoracic rotation.

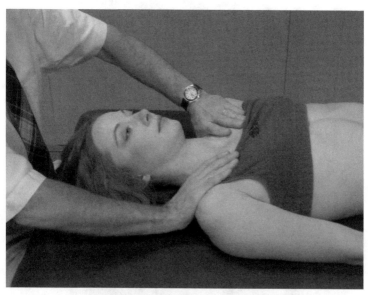

Cervicothoracic myofascial release

Indication: Thoracic paraspinal tension or restricted cervicothoracic fascia related to neck pain, headache, back pain, chest wall pain, edema, shortness of breath, and other problems.

Relative contraindications: Acute rib, sternum, or thoracic fracture.

Technique (seated or supine):

1. Place one hand across the sternal angle and the other hand across the vertebra with the most tension;
2. Indirect: Gently compress the hands together and follow any fascial give to its position of laxity, maintaining fascial laxity and following any tissue release until completed;
3. Direct: Gently move the cervicothoracic fascia into its flexion-extension, rotation, and sidebending restrictions and apply steady force until tissue give is completed;
4. Retest cervicothoracic motion.

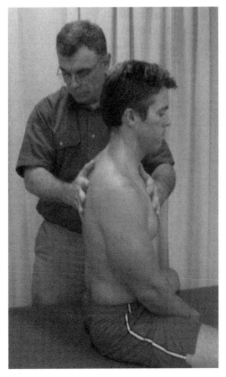

Seated cervicothoracic MFR

THORACIC OUTLET DIRECT MYOFASCIAL RELEASE

Indications: Tension or restriction associated with neck pain, back pain, thoracic outlet syndrome, or other problems.

Relative contraindications: Acute fracture, sprain, or dislocation; joint inflammation.

Technique (supine, lateral);

1. For scalene tension, use one hand to exert inferior and lateral traction with external rotation on the arm and your other hand to move the head into its restriction in rotation and sidebending away from the side of tension, applying steady stretch until tissue give is completed;
2. For trapezius or triceps tension, use one hand to stabilize the head and your other hand to move the arm into its traction and rotation restrictions, applying steady stretch until tissue give is completed;
3. For pectoralis tension, use one or both hands to move the arm into its abduction and extension barriers, applying steady stretch until tissue give is completed;
4. Retest for tension or restriction.

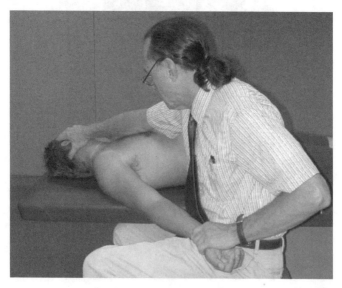

Scalene myofascial release

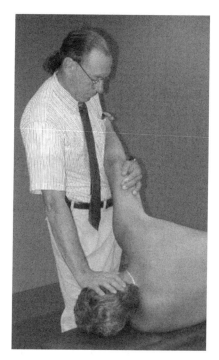

Trapezius/triceps myofascial release

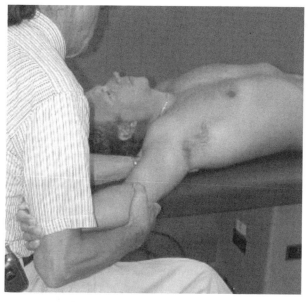

Pectoralis myofascial release

167

THORACIC MYOFASCIAL RELEASE

Indication: Restricted thoracic rotation related to back pain, chest wall pain, rib restriction, shoulder pain, and other problems.

Relative contraindications: Acute thoracic fracture.

Technique (supine):

1. Sitting at the head of the table, place your fingertips on the transverse processes of the restricted segment;

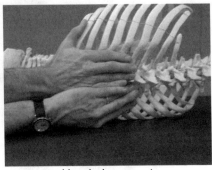

2. Indirect: Use your fingertips to gently move the segment to the position of rotation, sidebending, and flexion-extension laxity and follow any tissue release until completed;

Hand placement

3. Direct: Slowly move the segment into the rotation, sidebending, and flexion-extension restrictions and apply steady force until tissue give is completed;
4. Retest thoracic rotation.

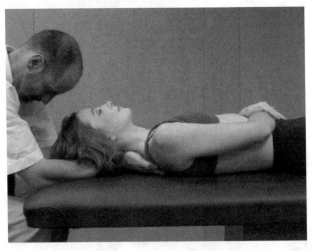

T4 myofascial release

THORACIC EXTENSION FACILITATED POSITIONAL RELEASE[1]

Indications: Thoracic extension somatic dysfunction associated with back pain, chest wall pain, and other problems.

Relative contraindications: Acute fracture, shoulder dislocation.

Technique (prone):

1. Place a pillow under the upper chest to decrease thoracic kyphosis if desired;
2. Have the patient turn the head toward the side of thoracic rotation;
3. Stand on the opposite side of thoracic rotation and palpate the paraspinal tension;
4. Slowly lift the shoulder on the side of thoracic rotation toward the paraspinal tension, adding compression or torsion until tension decreases;
5. Hold this position for 3–5 seconds until tension release is completed and slowly return the shoulder to the table;
6. Remove the pillow and retest thoracic rotation.

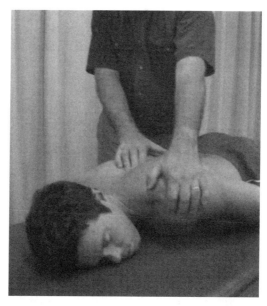

Thoracic extension FPR

THORACIC FLEXION FACILITATED POSITIONAL RELEASE[1]

Indications: Thoracic flexion somatic dysfunction associated with back pain, chest wall pain, and other problems.

Relative contraindications: Acute fracture.

Technique (seated):

1. Standing behind the patient, reach over the shoulder on the side of thoracic rotation and across the upper chest to hold the top of the other shoulder;
2. Palpate the paraspinal tension and ask the patient to sit up straight to reduce thoracic kyphosis;
3. Slowly flex the trunk until motion is felt at the restricted segment;
4. Rotate the shoulders toward the side of thoracic rotation until tension decreases and add compressive force through your axilla causing sidebending at the level being monitored;
5. Hold this position for 3–5 seconds until tension release is completed and slowly return the trunk to neutral;
6. Retest thoracic rotation.

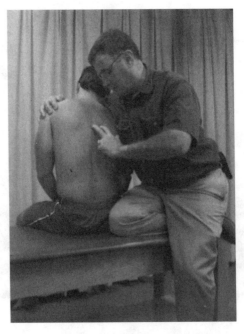

Thoracic flexion FPR for FRSright

STERNUM LIGAMENTOUS ARTICULAR STRAIN

Indication: Sternal fascial tension or restriction associated with chest wall pain and other problems.

Relative contraindications: Sternum fracture, rib fracture, costochondral subluxation.

Technique (supine):

1. Sit or stand at the head of the table and place the heel of your hand on the manubrium and fingertips at the xiphisternal junction;
2. Compress the sternum by pushing the manubrium posteriorly and inferiorly while pulling your fingertips posteriorly and superiorly;
3. Move the sternal fascia into its sidebending and rotation laxity;
4. Maintain sternal compression and fascial laxity, following any tissue release until completed;
5. Retest for fascial tension or restriction.

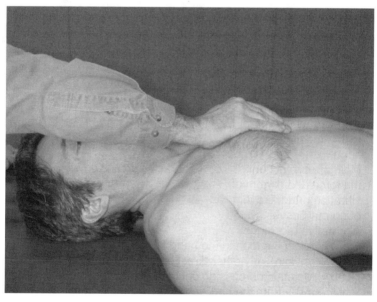

Sternum ligamentous articular strain

THORACIC PERCUSSION VIBRATOR

Indications: Thoracic somatic dysfunction associated with back pain, chest wall pain, anxiety, or other problems.

Relative contraindications: Acute thoracic or rib fracture, acute shoulder sprain or surgery, shoulder inflammation, pacemaker, defibrillator, thoracic cancer.

Technique (lateral):

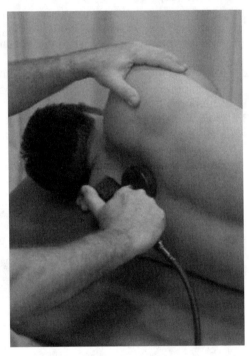

1. With the patient lying on the non-restricted side with knees and hips flexed, place your monitoring hand over the shoulder;
2. Place the vibrating percussion pad lightly on the involved thoracic spinous processes perpendicular to the surface, avoiding pad bouncing;
3. Alter pad speed, pressure, and angle until vibrations are palpated as strong by the monitoring hand;
4. Maintain contact until the force and rhythm of vibration returns to that of normal tissue;

Thoracic percussion vibrator

5. Alternative technique:
    a) Allow the monitoring hand to be pulled toward the pad, resisting any other direction of hand pull;
    b) Maintain percussion until the monitoring hand is pushed away from the pad;
6. Slowly release the monitoring hand and the percussion vibrator and retest tissue texture or motion.

172

Indication: Restricted thoracic rotation related to back pain, chest wall pain, shoulder pain, or other problems.

Relative contraindications: Joint inflammation, acute sprain, acute fracture, vertebral cancer, vertebral fusion (thrust only).

Technique:

1. Standing behind the seated patient, place your thenar eminence or thumb on the posterior transverse process(es);
2. Reach across the upper chest with your other hand and arm to control the patient's shoulders and trunk. For T1-4 restrictions hold the top of the head to induce cervical and upper thoracic motion;
3. Move the trunk or head into the rotation, sidebending, and flexion-extension restrictive barriers until you feel movement at the restricted segment(s);

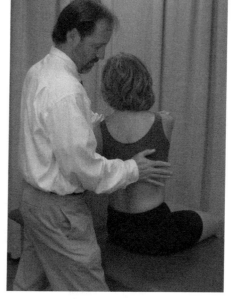

Muscle energy for T7 FRS right

4. Ask the patient to straighten out the trunk or head for 3-5 seconds against your equal resistance;
5. Slowly move the trunk or head to new restrictive barriers as you push anteriorly into the posterior transverse process(es);
6. Repeat 3-5 times or until thoracic mobility returns;
7. For T5-12 a thrust can be added if needed by a short and quick anterior push into the posterior transverse process(es) as you simultaneous move the trunk into its barriers;
8. Retest thoracic rotation.

THORACIC ARTICULATORY – SEATED

Indication: Restricted thoracic rotation related to back pain, chest wall pain, shoulder pain, or other problems.

Relative contraindications: Joint inflammation, joint hypermobility, acute sprain, acute fracture, vertebral cancer.

Technique (seated):

1. Stand behind the patient, place your thumb or thenar eminence on the posterior transverse process, and control the patient's shoulders with your other arm and hand;
2. Slowly move the patient into the position of laxity for flexion/extension, rotation, and sidebending;
3. In one smooth motion, slowly move the patient from the position of laxity into the restrictive barriers for flexion/extension, rotation, and sidebending while pushing anteriorly into the posterior transverse process;
4. Repeat 3-5 times or until joint mobility returns;
5. Retest vertebral rotation.

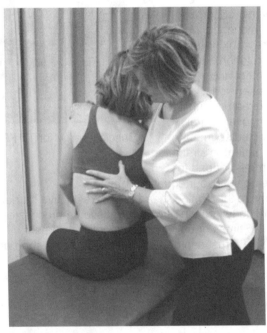

Articulatory for T7 FRS left

Indication: Restricted thoracic rotation or rib motion related to back pain, chest wall pain, shoulder pain, or other problems.

Relative contraindications: Joint inflammation, joint hypermobility, acute sprain, acute fracture, vertebral cancer.

Technique (supine):

1. Stand at the head of the patient whose hands are clasped behind the head;
2. Reach through the patients arms and hold the back of the rib cage;
3. Lift the upper back and place your bent knee under the restricted area;
4. Use your arms and body to slowly roll the patient backward over your knee while lifting the rib cage to mobilize restricted joints;
5. Repeat for other restricted areas;
6. Retest thoracic rotation.

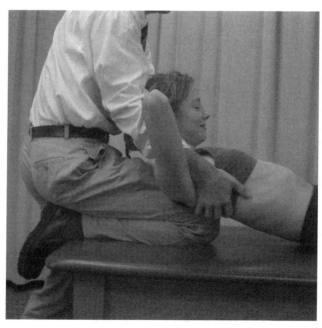

Supine thoracic articulatory

THORACIC THRUST – PRONE

Indication: Restricted thoracic rotation related to back pain, chest wall pain, shoulder pain, or other problems.

Relative contraindications: Joint inflammation, joint hypermobility, acute sprain, acute fracture, vertebral cancer, vertebral fusion.

Technique:

1. Stand on the side of thoracic rotation and place your hypothenar eminence on the posterior transverse process;
2. Place the thenar eminence of your other hand on the opposite transverse process of the segment above or below the one being treated;
3. Ask the patient to take a deep breath and follow exhalation with gentle anterior pressure from both hands;
4. At the end of exhalation apply a short quick thrust in an anterior direction with both hands;
5. Retest thoracic rotation.

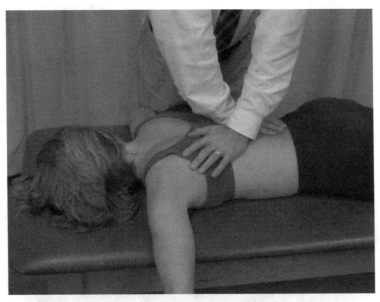

Prone thrust for T8 rotated right

THORACIC/RIB THRUST – SUPINE

Indication: Restricted thoracic rotation or rib motion (see p.195) related to back pain, chest wall pain, shoulder pain, or other problems.

Relative contraindications: Joint inflammation, joint hypermobility, acute sprain, acute fracture, costochondral subluxation, vertebral cancer, vertebral fusion, severe osteoporosis.

Technique:

1. Stand on the opposite side of thoracic rotation or rib restriction;
2. Cross the patient's arms with the elbows together and the arm on the side of thoracic rotation on top;
3. Reach your caudad arm across the patient and place the thenar eminence behind the posterior transverse process or rib angle;
4. Lean your epigastric area into the patient's crossed elbows;
5. Use your other hand to lift the patient's head and trunk until pressure from leaning on the elbows is felt by your thenar eminence;
6. Ask the patient to take a deep breath, lean into the elbows during exhalation, and at maximum exhalation quickly drop your abdomen onto the elbows to mobilize the joint;
7. Retest thoracic or rib motion.

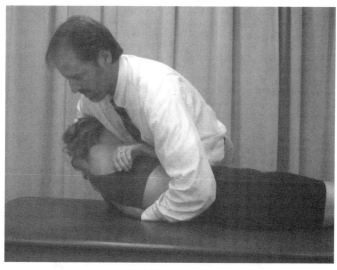

Supine thrust for T8 rotated right

THORACIC/RIB THRUST – SEATED

Indication: Restricted thoracic rotation or rib mobility (see p.195) related to back pain, chest wall pain, shoulder pain, or other problems.

Relative contraindications: Joint inflammation, joint hypermobility, acute sprain, acute fracture, vertebral cancer, vertebral fusion.

Technique:

1. Stand behind the patient whose hands are clasped behind the head;
2. Place your epigastric area behind the posterior transverse process or rib angle;
3. Reach under the patient's arms and hold the forearms;
4. Ask the patient to take a deep breath and during exhalation pull the elbows together, extend the trunk, and push your abdomen into the posterior transverse process or rib;
5. At maximal exhalation apply a short quick thrust with your abdomen into the posterior transverse process or rib angle;
6. Retest thoracic rotation or rib motion.

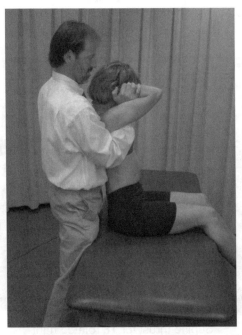

Thoracic/rib seated thrust

POSTERIOR THORACIC POSITION OF EASE

1. Lay face down with a pillow or two under your shoulder on the side of back pain;
2. Turn your head to the side of back pain and allow it to rest on the pillow;
3. If back pain is reduced, take a few deep breaths and rest in this position for 2-5 minutes;
4. Repeat 2-4 times a day or as needed for pain relief.

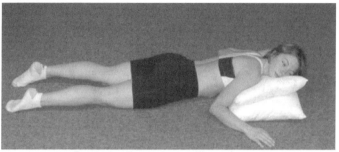
Posterior thoracic position of ease

ANTERIOR THORACIC POSITION OF EASE

1. Lie on your back with 2-3 pillows under the head;
2. If chest pain is reduced take a few deep breaths and rest in this position for 2-5 minutes. If pain is not reduced try adding or removing a pillow;
3. Repeat 2-4 times a day or as needed for pain relief.

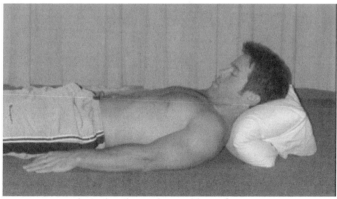
Anterior thoracic position of ease

THORACIC FLEXION/EXTENSION STRETCH[2]

1. Kneel with your arms straight and hands shoulder width apart;
2. Arch your back slowly upward while tucking the head and tailbone down;
3. Take a few deep breaths and stretch for 5-10 seconds;

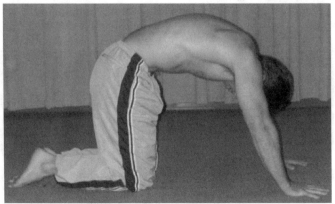

Thoracic flexion stretch

4. Arch your back slowly downward while curling the head and tailbone upward;
5. Take a few deep breaths and stretch for 5-10 seconds;
6. Repeat 3-5 times;
7. Do these stretches 1-4 times a day.

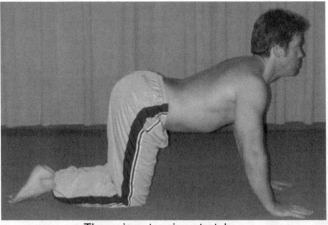

Thoracic extension stretch

THORACIC MOBILIZATION – SUPINE[2]

1. Lie on your back with knees bent and fingers locked behind the head;
2. Push your elbows together;
3. Use your arms to pull the head forward while simultaneously lifting the pelvis until a single vertebra touches the floor;
4. Rock the pelvis up and down to roll a vertebra over the floor until a mobilization is felt;
5. Repeat for other vertebrae if needed;
6. Do this mobilization up to twice a day.

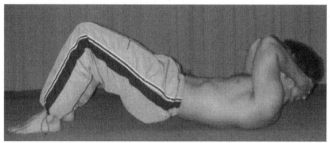

Thoracic mobilization - supine

THORACIC MOBILIZATION – KNEELING

1. Kneel with your arms straight and hands shoulder width;
2. Reach your left shoulder down toward the left hip as far as it will go;
3. Reach your right shoulder down toward the right hip as far as it will go;
4. Repeat 3-5 times;
5. Do this mobilization up to twice a day.

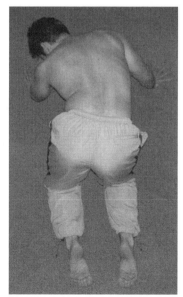

Thoracic mobilization – kneeling

THORACIC MOBILIZATION – STANDING[3]

1. Stand with arms hanging by your side;
2. Swing your arms to one side, allowing the back to follow as far as it will go;
3. Swing your arms to the other side, allowing the back to follow as far as it will go;
4. Repeat 3-5 times;
5. Clasp the hands behind your head;
6. Swing your arms to one side, allowing the head and upper back to follow as far as they will go;
7. Swing your arms to the other side, allowing the head and upper back to follow as far as they will go;
8. Repeat 3-5 times;
9. Do these mobilizations up to twice a day.

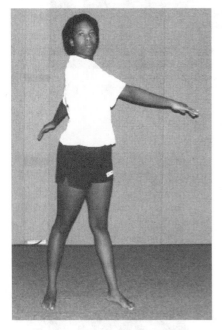
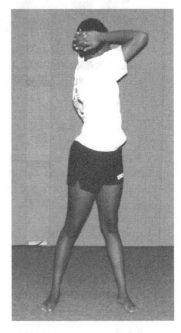

Lower thoracic mobilization   Mid-thoracic mobilization

REFERENCES

1. Adapted from Schiowitz S, DiGiovanna EL, Dowling DJ. *Chapter 64: Facilitated Positional Release* in Ward RC, Ed. *Foundations for Osteopathic Medicine 2nd Edition.* Lippincott Williams & Wilkins, Philadelphia, 2003.
2. Adapted from Kirk CE. *Biodynamics of self-administered manipulation.* 1977 AAO Yearbook, American Academy of Osteopathy, Colorado Springs, 1979.
3. Adapted from Steiner CS. *Tennis* elbow. Journal of the American Osteopathic Association 75(6):575-581. 1976.

THORACIC NOTES (cont.)

Chapter 8: RIB DIAGNOSIS AND TREATMENT

Diagnosis of Rib Somatic Dysfunction

Treatment of Rib Somatic Dysfunction

1. OMT

2. Exercises

3. Thermal therapy

Heat 20-30 minutes 4-6 times a day for tension or stiffness
Cold 15-20 minutes 4-6 times a day for pain relief

4. Stabilization

Prolotherapy for recurrent costochondral or chondrosternal subluxation

RIB ANGLE PALPATION

1. Flex and adduct one arm to move the scapula away from the posterior chest wall;
2. Palpate for symmetry and tenderness of the rib angles which become progressively lateral in the lower rib cage;
3. The following findings indicate the listed somatic dysfunctions (see p.191):
   a) Prominent rib angle = posterior rib subluxation;
   b) Depressed rib angle = anterior rib subluxation;
   c) Tender rib angle = elevated rib tender point, rib subluxation, or key rib.

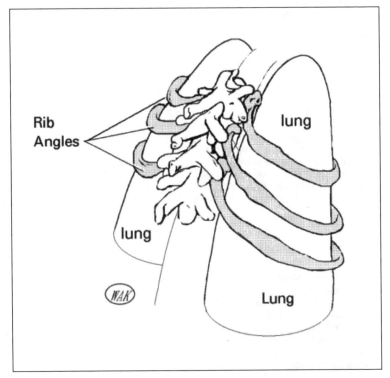

A rib angle is the posterior prominence

(William A. Kuchera, DO, FAAO)

1. Palpate for posterior (elevated) rib tender points at the following locations:

   a) **Posterior rib 1** – lateral shaft anterior to trapezius muscle;
   b) **Posterior ribs 2-7** – rib angles with scapula rotated away by flexing and adducting arm;
   c) **Posterior ribs 8-10** – rib angles which are more lateral with each lower rib.

2. Palpate for anterior (depressed) rib tender points at the following locations:

   a) **Anterior rib 1** – inferior to medial clavicle, lateral to sternum;
   b) **Anterior rib 2** – rib shaft in mid-clavicular line;
   c) **Anterior ribs 3-10** – rib shaft in anterior axillary line or mid-axillary line.

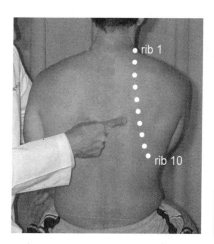 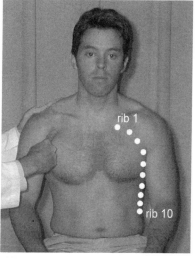

| Posterior rib tender points (right PT8 shown) | Anterior rib tender points (pectoralis minor palpation shown) |

189

RIB MOTION TESTING

1. Let your fingers rest gently on the shafts of the ribs being assessed:
   Rib 1 – first fingers at the base of the lateral neck just anterior to the trapezius muscle;
   Ribs 2-5 – fingers on anteromedial shafts along the sternum;
   Ribs 6-10 – fingers on the lateral shafts in the mid-axillary line;
   Ribs 11-12 – first and second fingers on shafts posteriorly;
2. Ask the patient to breathe deeply in and out and passively follow rib motion;
3. Restricted rib exhalation = inhalation somatic dysfunction;
4. Restricted rib inhalation = exhalation somatic dysfunction.

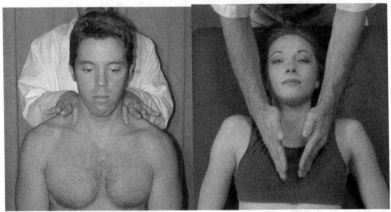

Rib 1   Ribs 2-5

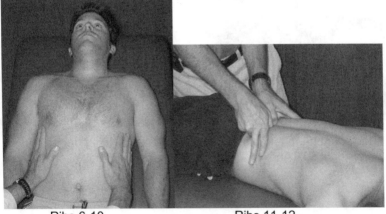

Ribs 6-10   Ribs 11-12

Somatic Dysfunction	Diagnostic Finding	Key Rib[1]
Posterior tender point	tenderness at rib angle	most tender rib
Anterior tender point	tenderness on rib shaft at anterior or mid-axillary line	most tender rib
Posterior subluxation	prominent rib angle	
Anterior subluxation	anterior rib angle	
Inhalation somatic dysfunction[2]	restricted exhalation	inferior rib
Exhalation somatic dysfunction[2]	restricted inhalation	superior rib

[1]The key rib is the rib in a group somatic dysfunction which can be treated first to allow resolution of associated rib somatic dysfunctions.
[2]For rib 1, inhalation somatic dysfunction is termed an elevated 1st rib and exhalation somatic dysfunction is termed a depressed 1st rib.

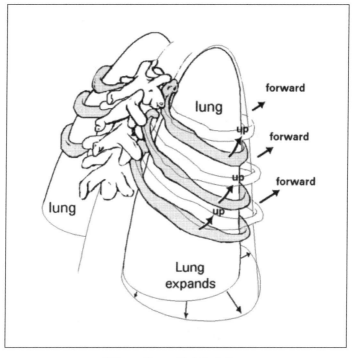

Rib motion with inhalation

(William A. Kuchera, DO, FAAO)

RIB 1 COUNTERSTRAIN

Indication: Posterior (elevated) rib 1 tender point associated with shoulder pain, neck pain, headache, thoracic outlet syndrome, and other problems.

Relative contraindications: Acute cervical fracture.

Technique (seated):

1. Locate the tender point on the shaft of the first rib at the lower neck just anterior to the upper trapezius muscle, labeling it 10/10;
2. Place your foot on the table on the side of the tender point and drape the patient's arm over your thigh;
3. Lean the patient into your thigh, sidebend the head toward the tender point, and retest for tenderness;
4. Fine tune this position with slight cervical extension and rotation until tenderness is 2/10 or less;
5. Hold the position of relief for 90 seconds;
6. Slowly and passively return to neutral and retest for tenderness.

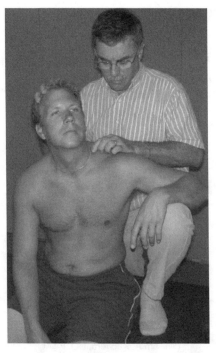

Elevated left 1st rib counterstrain

RIB 1 ARTICULATORY

Indication: Restricted rib 1 exhalation associated with neck pain, headache, thoracic outlet syndrome, shoulder pain, or other problems.

Relative contraindications: Acute sprain or fracture, rib 1 hypermobility, dizziness or nausea with cervical rotation.

Technique (seated):

1. Hold the patient's head with one hand and place the first metacarpal-phalangeal joint of your other hand on the posterior aspect of the elevated first rib;
2. Push the rib inferomedially while you slowly move the head into sidebending away from the rib, extension, sidebending toward the rib, and flexion in one smooth motion;
3. Repeat 3–5 times or until rib mobility returns;
4. Retest rib 1 motion.

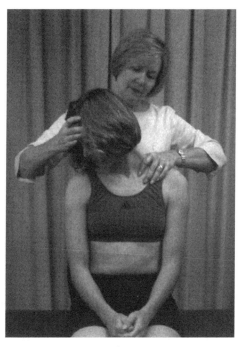

Elevated left 1ˢᵗ rib articulatory

RIB 1 MUSCLE ENERGY/THRUST – SUPINE

Indication: Restricted first rib exhalation associated with neck pain, headache, thoracic outlet syndrome, shoulder pain, or other problems.

Relative contraindications: Acute cervical sprain or fracture, undiagnosed cervical radiculopathy, vertebral cancer, rib 1 hypermobility (thrust only).

Technique:

1. Hold the occiput in your palms and place your first metacarpal-phalangeal (MCP) joint at the posterolateral aspect of the elevated first rib with that arm pointing toward the opposite axilla;
2. Push the rib in an anteromedial and inferior direction as you sidebend the head around your MCP joint and rotate the head to the opposite side;
3. Ask the patient to straighten the head for 3-5 seconds against your equal resistance;
4. Repeat 3-5 times or until rib mobilization occurs;
5. If needed, apply a short and quick thrust into the rib toward the opposite axilla;
6. Retest rib 1 motion.

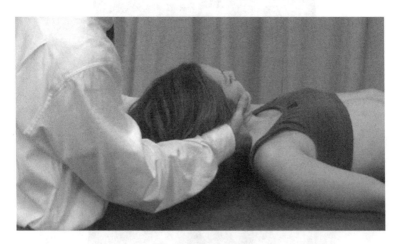

Supine muscle energy/thrust for elevated right first rib

Indication: Restricted first rib exhalation associated with neck pain, headache, thoracic outlet syndrome, shoulder pain, or other problems.

Relative contraindications: Acute cervical sprain or fracture, rib 1 hypermobility, undiagnosed cervical radiculopathy, vertebral cancer.

Technique:

1. Stand at the head of the prone patient whose chin is on the table;
2. Reach across the head and place your thenar or hypothenar eminence on the posterior aspect of the elevated first rib, pushing toward the ASIS on the same side;
3. Reach under your arm with the other hand and slowly roll the head into a sidebending restrictive barrier away from the elevated rib;
4. Apply a short quick thrust onto the rib toward the ipsilateral ASIS;
5. Retest first rib motion.

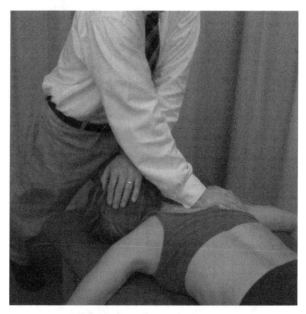

Prone thrust for elevated right first rib

RIB 1 THRUST – SEATED

Indication: Restricted first rib exhalation associated with neck pain, headache, thoracic outlet syndrome, shoulder pain, or other problems.

Relative contraindications: Acute sprain or fracture, rib 1 hypermobility, undiagnosed cervical radiculopathy, vertebral cancer.

Technique:

1. Place your first metacarpal-phalangeal joint on the posterolateral aspect of the elevated first rib, hold the patient's head with your other hand, and lean the patient away from the elevated rib by draping his or her arm over your thigh with your foot on the table;
2. Push the rib in an anteromedial and inferior direction, sidebend the head toward the elevated rib, lean the patient farther over your thigh, and apply a short quick thrust into the rib toward the opposite axilla;
3. Retest rib 1 motion.

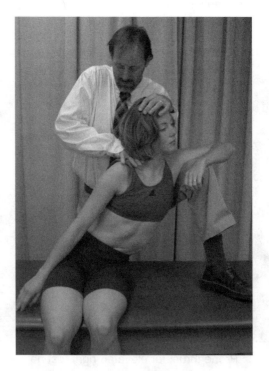

Seated thrust for elevated right first rib

POSTERIOR RIB 2-10 COUNTERSTRAIN

Indication: Posterior rib tender point associated with back pain, chest wall pain, and other problems.

Relative contraindications: Acute thoracic or rib sprain or fracture.

Technique (seated):

1. Locate the tender point on the posterior rib angle, labeling it 10/10;
2. Place your foot on the table to the side of the tender point and drape the patient's arm over your thigh;
3. Lean the patient into your thigh and retest for tenderness;
4. Fine tune this position with more sidebending and slight trunk rotation until tenderness is 2/10 or less;
5. Hold the position of relief for 90 seconds;
6. Slowly and passively return to neutral and retest for tenderness.

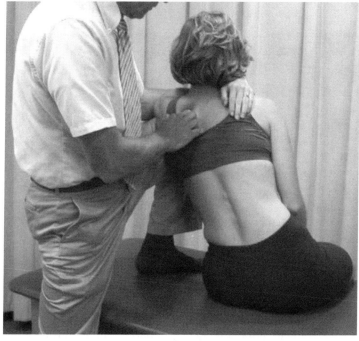

Posterior left 3rd rib counterstrain

ANTERIOR RIB 1-2 COUNTERSTRAIN

Indication: Anterior rib 1 or 2 tender point associated with chest wall pain, neck pain, and other problems.

Relative contraindications: Acute cervical or rib fracture or dislocation.

Technique (supine):

1. Locate the tender point inferior to the clavicle and just lateral to the sternum (rib 1) or in the mid-clavicular line (rib 2), labeling it 10/10;
2. Flex the head, rotate and sidebend it toward the tender point, and retest for tenderness;
3. Fine tune this position with slight changes in flexion, sidebending, and rotation until tenderness is 2/10 or less;
4. Hold the position of relief for 90 seconds;
5. Slowly and passively return the head to neutral and retest for tenderness.

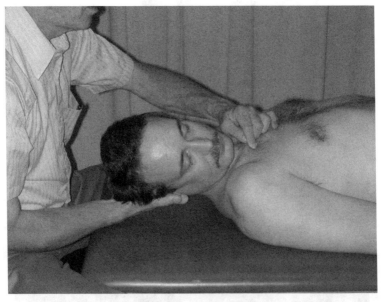

Right anterior rib 1 tender point and treatment position

ANTERIOR RIB 3–10 COUNTERSTRAIN

Indication: Anterior rib tender point associated with chest wall pain and other problems.

Relative contraindications: Acute thoracic or rib sprain or fracture.

Technique (seated):

1. Locate the anterior rib tender point, labeling 10/10;
2. Place your foot on the table to the opposite side of the tender point and drape the patient's arm over your thigh;
3. Lean the patient into your thigh and retest for tenderness;
4. Fine tune this position with more sidebending and slight trunk rotation until tenderness is 2/10 or less;
5. Hold the position of relief for 90 seconds;
6. Slowly and passively return to neutral and retest for tenderness.

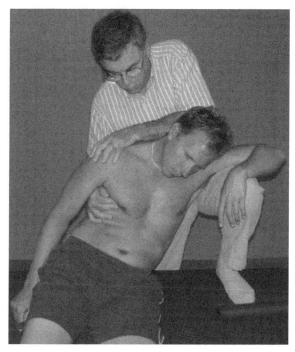

Anterior right 6th rib counterstrain

Anterior right 6th rib counterstrain

RIB MYOFASCIAL RELEASE

Indication: Rib somatic dysfunction related to back pain, chest wall pain, and other problems.

Relative contraindications: Acute rib fracture.

Technique (seated or supine):

1. Hold the involved rib angle with two fingers of one hand and the anterior rib with two fingers of your other hand, placing your thumbs along the lateral rib;
2. Apply gentle anterior-posterior compression between your hands until any tissue give is completed;
3. Apply gentle lateral traction to the entire rib and follow any tissue release until completed;
4. Slowly release the rib and retest rib motion.

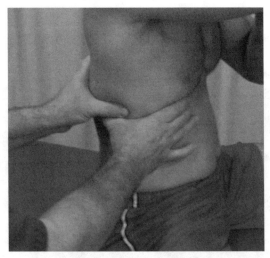

Rib myofascial release

RIB MYOFASCIAL RELEASE USING SHOULDER

Indication: Rib restriction or tender point related to back pain, chest wall pain, and other problems.

Relative contraindications: Acute rib fracture, acute shoulder sprain, shoulder joint inflammation.

Technique (supine):

1. Sitting at the head of the table, reach behind the shoulder with one hand and pull the involved rib angle superiorly;
2. Grasp the proximal forearm and slowly abduct the arm while maintaining shoulder internal rotation and superior pull on the rib, holding steady force at any restriction until tissue give is completed;
3. Slowly externally rotate the arm and move it into additional abduction while maintaining superior pull on the rib, holding steady force at any restriction until tissue give is completed;
4. Slowly adduct the arm while maintaining arm external rotation and superior pull on the rib, holding steady force at any restriction until tissue give is completed and placing the arm at the patient's side;
5. Maintaining superior pull on the rib, move your other hand from the forearm to the shoulder and repetitively compress the shoulder toward the rib for 10 to 20 seconds or until rib movement occurs;
6. Slowly return the arm to the table and retest rib motion.

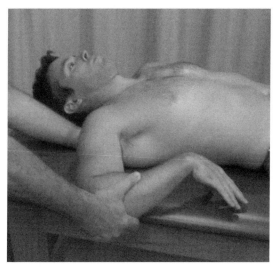

Abduction

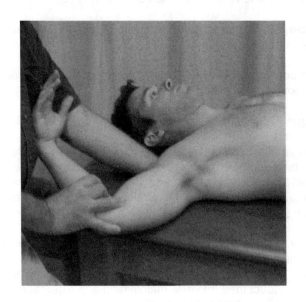

External rotation

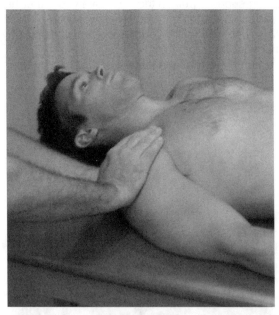

Compression

FOCAL INHIBITION FACILITATED OSCILLATORY RELEASE

Indication: Tissue tension or tenderness associated with pain, restricted mobility, or other problems.

Relative contraindications: Acute fracture, significant patient guarding.

Technique (supine, prone, lateral, seated):

1. Place one or two fingertips on the target tissue;
2. Use your other hand to apply positional stretch by moving the body or skin away from the target tissue;
3. Initiate oscillatory force through the fingertips into the target tissue by rhythmically moving your forearm;
4. Continue oscillation until tension is reduced.

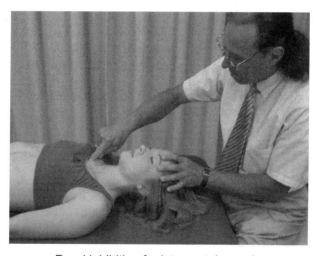

Focal inhibition for intercostal muscle

RIB PERCUSSION VIBRATOR

Indication: Rib somatic dysfunction associated with chest wall pain, back pain, shortness of breath, cough, and other problems.

Contraindications: Acute rib fracture or costochondral separation, pacemaker, defibrillator, rib cancer, pregnancy.

Technique (supine):

1. Place your monitoring hand on the left mid-axillary line at the level of rib somatic dysfunction;
2. Place the vibrating percussion pad lightly on a depression in the right mid-axillary line at the level of rib somatic dysfunction;
3. Alter pad speed, pressure, and angle until vibrations are palpated as strong by the monitoring hand;
4. Maintain contact until the force and rhythm of vibration returns to that of normal tissue;
5. Alternative technique:
    a) Allow the monitoring hand to be pulled toward the pad, resisting any other direction of hand pull;
    b) Maintain percussion until the monitoring hand is pushed away from the pad;
6. Slowly release the monitoring hand and the percussion vibrator and retest for rib somatic dysfunction.

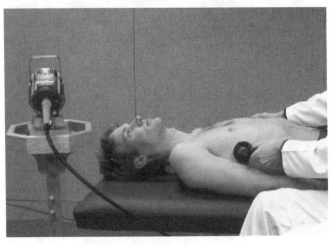

Rib 6 percussion vibrator

Indication: Anterior or posterior rib subluxation associated with chest wall pain, back pain, shoulder pain, and other problems.

Relative contraindications: Severe osteoporosis, acute rib fracture, acute costochondral subluxation, vertebral or rib cancer.

Technique (seated):

1. Stand behind the patient and use your thenar eminence or thumb to push the involved rib as follows:
   Posterior subluxation – push the rib angle anteromedially;
   Anterior subluxation – push the costotransverse articulation posterolaterally;
2. Ask the patient to push the flexed elbow as follows for 3-5 seconds against your equal resistance:
   Posterior subluxation – the patient pushes the elbow medially;
   Anterior subluxation – the patient pushes the elbow laterally;
3. During relaxation maintain pressure on the rib until give stops;
4. Repeat 3-5 times or until rib symmetry returns;
5. Retest rib angle symmetry.

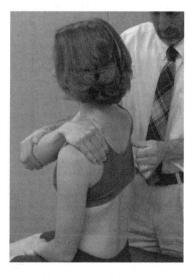 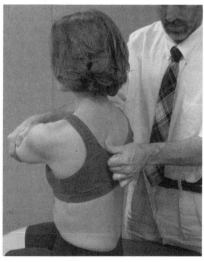

Posterior subluxation   Anterior subluxation

RIB INHALATION MUSCLE ENERGY

Indication: Rib exhalation restriction associated with chest wall pain, back pain, shoulder pain, and other problems.

Relative contraindications: Severe osteoporosis, acute rib fracture, acute costochondral subluxation, vertebral or rib cancer.

Technique (supine):

1. Sit or stand at the head of the supine patient;
2. Use your palm, thumb, or fingers to push inferiorly on the shaft of the inferior rib in the group:
   Ribs 2-5 – push inferiorly on rib shaft in the anterior axillary line. Avoid breast contact for a female patient by pushing on the medial aspect of the rib near the sternum or onto her hand placed on the rib shaft (shown below);
   Ribs 6-10 – push inferiorly on rib shaft in the mid-axillary line;
3. Use your other hand to flex and sidebend the neck and thorax until inferior motion is felt at the inferior rib in the group;
4. Ask the patient to inhale deeply while you resist superior rib movement;
5. During exhalation push the rib more inferiorly as you flex and sidebend the neck and thorax a little farther;
6. Repeat 3-5 times or until rib motion returns;
7. Retest rib motion.

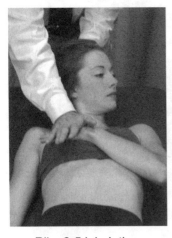
Ribs 2-5 inhalation

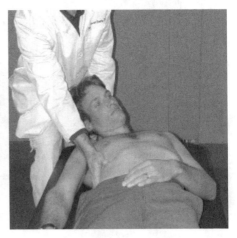
Ribs 6-10 inhalation

RIB EXHALATION MUSCLE ENERGY

Indication: Rib inhalation restriction associated with chest wall pain, back pain, shoulder pain, and other problems.

Relative contraindications: Severe osteoporosis, acute rib fracture, acute costochondral subluxation, vertebral or rib cancer.

Technique (supine):

1. Sit on the side of the rib restriction and use the fingers of one hand to pull inferiorly on the rib angle of the superior rib in the group;
2. Ask the patient to push for 3-5 seconds against your equal resistance:
   > Rib 2 – flex the head which is rotated slightly away (posterior scalene contraction);
   > Ribs 3-5 – push the elbow of the abducted arm across the chest (pectoralis minor contraction);
   > Ribs 6-10 – push the abducted arm down toward the side (serratus anterior contraction);
3. Pull the rib angle inferiorly to a new barrier;
4. Repeat 3-5 times or until rib motion returns;
5. Retest rib motion.

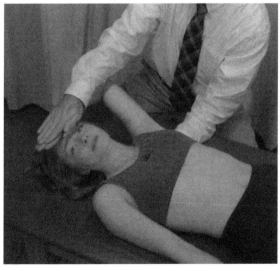

Muscle energy for rib 2 exhalation

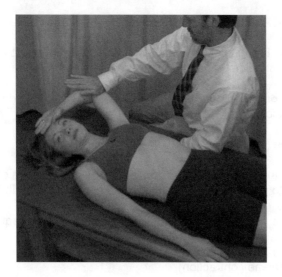
Muscle energy for ribs 3-5

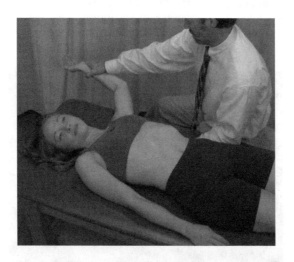
Muscle energy for ribs 6-10

Indication: Rib 11 or 12 restriction associated with back pain, chest wall pain, and other problems.

Relative contraindications: Acute rib fracture, vertebral or rib cancer.

Technique (prone):

1. Stand on the opposite side of the restricted rib and place your thumb on the inferior aspect of the rib to create a fulcrum:
   Inhalation restriction – thumb on rib shaft;
   Exhalation restriction – thumb on costotransverse articulation;
2. Pull the ASIS posteriorly on the side of rib restriction to stretch the quadratus lumborum muscle until give stops;
3. Ask the patient to push the hip toward the table for 3-5 seconds against your equal resistance;
4. During relaxation slowly pull the ASIS posteriorly until tissue give stops;
5. Repeat 3-5 times or until rib motion returns;
6. Retest rib motion.

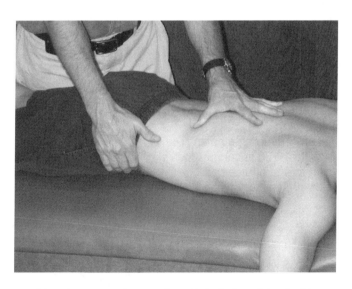

Muscle energy for restricted inhalation right rib 11

POSTERIOR RIB POSITION OF EASE

1. Sit with your arm on the side of back pain resting on a table or counter;
2. Lean toward the table until pain is reduced;
3. If comfortable, take a few deep breaths and rest in this position for 2-5 minutes;
4. Slowly sit back up and let the arm drop to your side;
5. Repeat 2-4 times a day or as needed for pain relief.

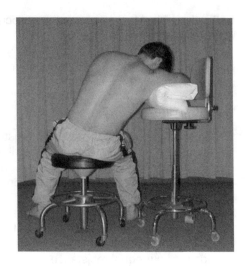

Position for right posterior rib

LATISSIMUS STRETCH

1. Stand with your feet shoulder width apart;
2. Place one arm behind your head;
3. With the other hand grasp the elbow and slowly lean your trunk away from the arm behind the head;
4. Take a few deep breaths and stretch for 10-20 seconds;
5. Repeat for the other side;
6. Do this stretch 1-4 times a day.

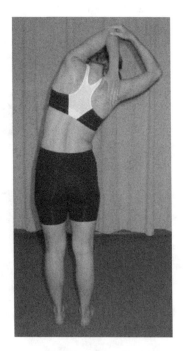

Left latissimus stretch

ANTERIOR RIB POSITION OF EASE

1. Sit with your arm on the pain free side resting on a table or counter;
2. Lean toward the table until pain is reduced;
3. If comfortable, rest in this position for 2-5 minutes;
4. Slowly sit back up and let the arm fall to your side;
5. Repeat 2-4 times a day or as needed for pain relief.

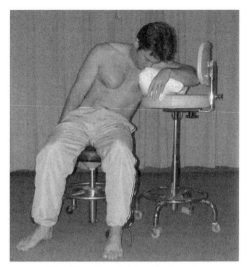

Position for right anterior rib

PECTORAL STRETCH

1. Kneel with your hands flat on the floor slightly in front of your head;
2. Squat back toward your heels as far as you can while keeping the arms straight and letting the chest drop down toward the floor;
3. Take a few deep breaths and stretch for 10-20 seconds;
4. Do this stretch 1-4 times a day.

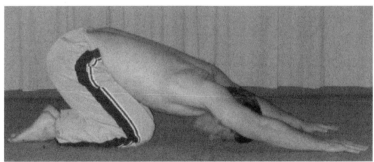

Pectoral stretch

RIB 1 MOBILIZATION

1. Sit with one hand firmly holding the top of the other shoulder at the base of the neck on the side of the restricted rib;
2. Slowly move your head in a circle, bending toward the hand, forward, away from the hand, backward, and toward the hand again. Stop if dizziness, nausea, or blurred vision occurs;
3. Repeat until first rib movement occurs;
4. Do this mobilization up to twice a day.

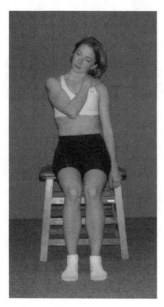

Left 1st rib mobilization

RIB MOBILIZATION

1. Lie on your back with knees bent and fingers locked behind the head;
2. Push your elbows together and roll the arms to one side;
3. Use your arms to pull the head forward while simultaneously lifting the pelvis until a single rib touches the floor;
4. Rock the pelvis up and down to roll the rib over the floor until a mobilization is felt;
5. Repeat for other ribs if needed;
6. Do this mobilization up to twice a day.

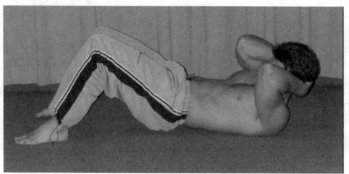

Rib mobilization

RIB NOTES (cont.)

RIB NOTES (cont.)

Chapter 9: CERVICAL DIAGNOSIS AND TREATMENT

Diagnosis of Cervical Somatic Dysfunction

1. Screening:
   a) Cervical range of motion – p.218
   b) Posterior cervical palpation – p.219
   c) Anterior cervical palpation – p.220
2. Typical cervical motion testing
   a) Sidebending testing – p.221
   b) Translation testing – p.222
3. Atlantoaxial motion testing – p.244
4. Occipitoatlantal motion testing – p.245
5. Cervical somatic dysfunction – pp.223-224
6. Neurological exam before treatment
   a) Upper extremity strength, deep tendon reflexes, sensation
   b) Cervical compression test – p.225
   c) Vertebral artery challenge test – p.225

Treatment of Cervical Somatic Dysfunction

1. OMT

Suboccipital inhibition – p.226
Cervical kneading – p.227
Cervical stretching – p.228
Scalene ligamentous articular strain – pp.229-230
Posterior C2-C7 counterstrain – p.231
Anterior C1 counterstrain – p.232
Anterior C2-C7 counterstrain – p.233
Cervicothoracic myofascial release – see p.164
Cervicothoracic myofascial release, seated – see p.165
Cervical myofascial release – p.234
Cervical ligamentous articular strain – p.235
Occipitoatlantal myofascial release – p.236

Cervical soft tissue facilitated positional release – p.237
Suboccipital facilitated oscillatory release – p.238
Cervical sidebending muscle energy/thrust – p.239
Cervical rotation muscle energy/thrust – p.240
Cervical articulatory, seated – p.241
Cervical sidebending articulatory – p.242
Cervical rotation articulatory – p.243
Atlantoaxial muscle energy/thrust – p.244
Occipitoatlantal muscle energy/thrust – p.245

2. Exercises

Posterior cervical position of ease – p.246
Cervical extensor stretch – p.246
Trapezius stretch – p.247
Levator stretch – p.247
Scalene position of ease – p.248
Scalene stretch – p.248

Sternocleidomastoid position of ease – p.249
Sternocleidomastoid stretch – p.249
Cervical joint position of ease – p.250
Cervical sidebending mobilization – p.250

3. Thermal therapy
   Heat 20-30 minutes 4-6 times a day for tension or stiffness
   Cold 15-20 minutes 4-6 times a day for pain relief

4. Stabilization – prolotherapy for ligamentous laxity.

CERVICAL RANGE OF MOTION

1. With the patient seated, observe for the following normal ranges of active (patient induced) motion[1]:
   a) Flexion ≥ 50°
   b) Extension ≥ 60°
   c) Rotation ≥ 80°
   d) Sidebending ≥ 45°
2. With the patient seated or supine, test the following ranges of passive (physician induced) motion which are normally equal to or greater than active motion:
   a) Flexion
   b) Extension
   c) Rotation
   d) Sidebending
3. Restricted active and passive motion = somatic dysfunction or anatomical restriction;
4. Restricted active and normal passive motion = possible muscle weakness, fatigue, inhibition, or guarding;
5. Restricted passive and normal active motion = muscle guarding.

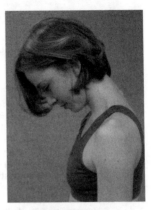

Active flexion

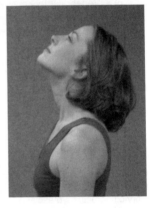

Active extension

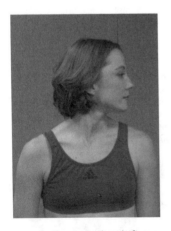

Active rotation left

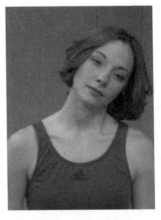

Active sidebending left

POSTERIOR CERVICAL PALPATION

1. Palpate for tension and tenderness in the paraspinal musculature;
2. Tender point locations:

   Posterior C2-C7 midline – spinous processes;
   Posterior C2-C7 lateral – posterior aspect of articular pillar at facet joint.

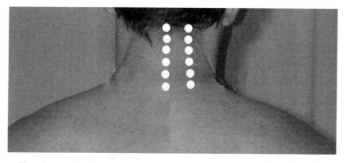

Tender point locations (lateral points are on both sides)

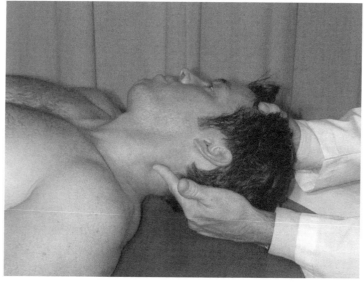

Palpation of left PC3 lateral tender point

ANTERIOR CERVICAL PALPATION

1. Palpate for tension and tenderness in the scalene and sternocleidomastoid muscles;
2. Palpate for the following tender points:

    Anterior C1 – tip of C1 transverse process or posterior mandible angle;
    Anterior C2-C6 – anterior aspect of articular pillar at facet joints;
    Anterior C7 – just superior to medial clavicle.

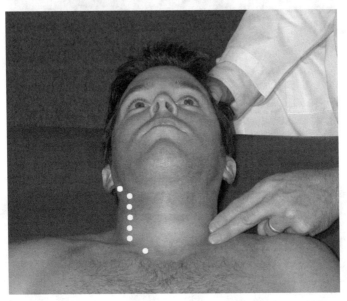

Palpation of scalene muscles (tender points indicated)

CERVICAL SEGMENTAL MOTION TESTING

1. With the patient supine, gently hold the occiput in your palms and place your fingertips on the lateral aspects of the articular pillars of the segment with facet joint fullness;
2. Induce segmental sidebending by simultaneously bending the head to one side and pushing medially into the articular pillar on that side, comparing to the other side to identify laxity and restriction;
3. Induce segmental rotation by pushing anteriorly into the articular pillar on one side, comparing to the other side to identify laxity and restriction;
4. If restricted, retest sidebending or rotation in cervical flexion (head lifted) and extension (articular pillars lifted);
5. Restricted sidebending or rotation left = sidebending and rotation right somatic dysfunction;
Restricted sidebending or rotation right = sidebending and rotation left somatic dysfunction;
5. Restriction worse in flexion = flexion restriction, extension somatic dysfunction;
Restriction worse in extension = extension restriction, flexion somatic dysfunction.

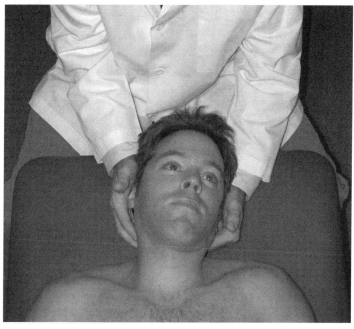

Testing C3 sidebending left

CERVICAL TRANSLATION TESTING

1. With the patient supine, gently hold the head in your palms and place your fingertips on the lateral aspects of the articular pillars of the segment being tested (occiput for occipitoatlantal joints);
2. Move the head and segment being tested laterally to one side to induce sidebending to the other side;
3. Compare to translation toward the other side to identify sidebending restriction;
4. If restricted, retest translation in cervical flexion (head lifted) and extension (articular pillars lifted);
5. Restricted translation left = restricted sidebending right = sidebending left somatic dysfunction;
    Restricted translation right = restricted sidebending left = sidebending right somatic dysfunction;
6. Restriction worse in flexion = flexion restriction, extension somatic dysfunction;
    Restriction worse in extension = extension restriction, flexion somatic dysfunction.

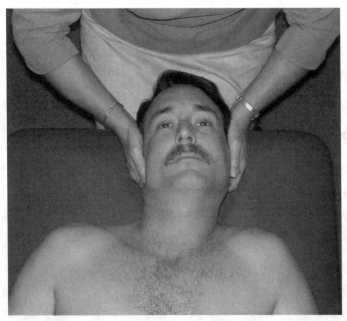

Testing OA translation left/sidebending right

CERVICAL SOMATIC DYSFUNCTION

Somatic Dysfunction[1]	Diagnostic Finding
Posterior tender point	tenderness at posterior articular pillar
Anterior tender point	tenderness at anterior articular pillar
C2-7 F Sx Rx	restricted C2-7 sidebending y and rotation y worse in extension
C2-7 E Sx Rx	restricted C2-7 sidebending y and rotation y worse in flexion
AA Rx	restricted C1 rotation y
OA F Sx Ry	restricted occiput sidebending y and rotation x worse in extension
OA E Sx Ry	restricted occiput sidebending y and rotation x worse in flexion

[1]Abbreviations: F = flexion; E = extension; S = sidebending; R = rotation; x = right or left; y = left or right (opposite x); AA = atlantoaxial; OA = occipitoatlantal.

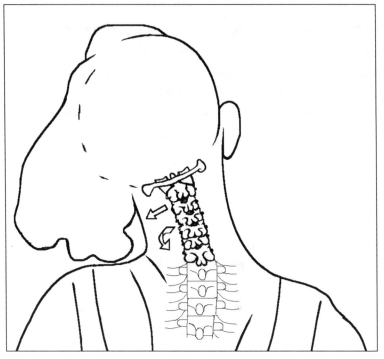

C2-7 sidebending left is accompanied by rotation left

(drawing by William A. Kuchera, DO, FAAO)

CERVICAL COMPRESSION TEST

Indication: Neck pain radiating to the arm or associated with arm numbness, tingling, or weakness.

1. With the patient seated or supine, place your hands on top of the head and push firmly in an inferior direction without flexing or extending the neck;
2. Reproduction or exacerbation of arm pain, numbness, or tingling indicates possible cervical neuritis as cause for arm symptoms.

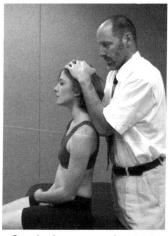

Cervical compression test

VERTEBRAL ARTERY CHALLENGE TEST

Indication: Screening for vertebral artery insufficiency before cervical manipulation.

1. With the patient seated or supine, gently rotate and extend the head as far as possible while observing the eyes and asking the patient to report any symptoms;
2. Maintain this position for 20 seconds unless   symptoms develop;
3. Dizziness, nausea, sweating, or nystagmus in this position indicates possible vertebral artery insufficiency;
4. If no symptoms develop, repeat with rotation to the other side.

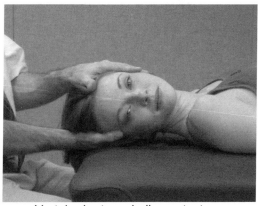

Vertebral artery challenge test

SUBOCCIPITAL INHIBITION

Indications: Suboccipital muscle tension association with neck pain, headache, respiratory congestion, visceral dysfunction, and other problems.

Relative contraindications: Atlantoaxial instability, meningismus.

Technique (supine):

1. Hold the occiput in your palms and align your fingertips inferior to the inion;
2. Straighten your fingers to press the fingertips into the suboccipital muscles;
3. Hold this position until the muscles relax and the head drops into your palms;
4. Retest for suboccipital muscle tension.

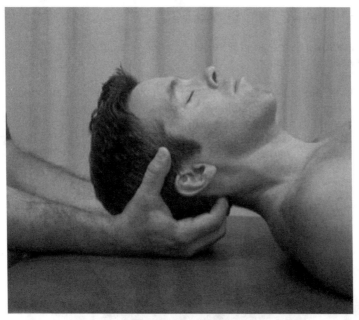

Suboccipital inhibition

CERVICAL KNEADING

Indications: Cervical paraspinal muscle tension associated with neck pain, headache, and other problems.

Relative contraindications: Meningismus.

Technique (supine):

1. Standing on the opposite side of muscle tension, place your cephalad hand on the forehead and use your other hand to grasp the paraspinal musculature lateral to the spinous processes;
2. Slowly pull the tense muscles anteriorly without sliding over the skin, resisting head rotation with your cephalad hand;
3. Repeat kneading until tension is reduced;
4. Repeat for the other side if needed.

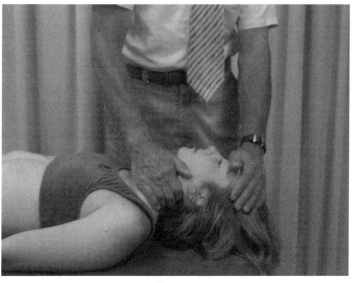

Cervical kneading

CERVICAL STRETCHING

Indications: Posterior cervical muscle tension associated with neck pain, headache, upper back pain, and other problems.

Relative contraindications: Acute strain and sprain, acute fracture, meningismus.

Technique (supine):

1. Cross your wrists under the occiput, place your palms downward on top of the shoulders, and slowly stand up to flex the neck as far as it will comfortably go. Alternative technique: Hold the occiput in your palms and slowly flex the neck as far as it will comfortably go;
2. Maintain gentle force at the flexion barrier until tissue give is completed;
3. Slowly lower the head to the table and retest for muscle tension.

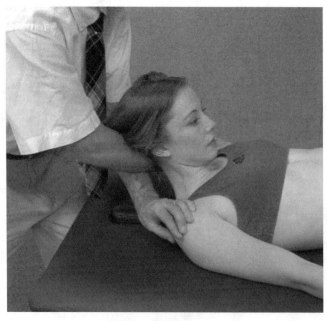

Cervical stretching

SCALENE LIGAMENTOUS ARTICULAR STRAIN

Indication: Scalene tension associated with neck pain, headache, facial pain, thoracic outlet syndrome, and other problems.

Relative contraindications: Supraclavicular mass.

Technique (supine):

1. Sit at the head of the table and place your thumb pads in the supraclavicular fossa just lateral to the sternocleidomastoid muscles;
2. Gently push your thumbs inferiorly into the anterior scalene muscles;
3. Maintain inferior pressure until tissue give is completed;
4. Gently pull your thumbs laterally, maintaining inferior and lateral pressure until tissue give is completed;
5. Place your thumb pads just posterior to the anterior scalene position and gently push inferiorly and medially into the middle and posterior scalene muscles;
6. Maintain inferior and medial pressure until tissue give is completed;
7. Retest for scalene tension.

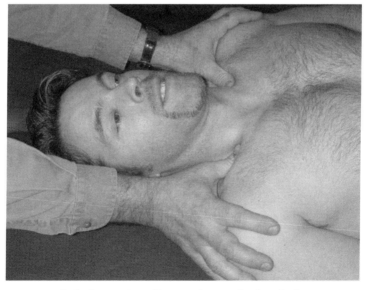

Anterior scalene ligamentous articular strain

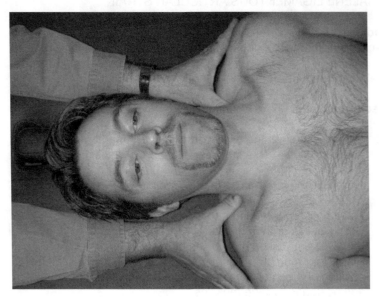

Middle and posterior scalene ligamentous articular strain

POSTERIOR C2-C7 COUNTERSTRAIN

Indication: Posterior C2-C7 tender point associated with neck pain, headache, and other problems.

Relative contraindications: Acute fracture or dislocation, vertebrobasilar insufficiency.

Technique (supine):

1. Locate the tender point on the spinous process or articular pillar, labeling it 10/10 (see p.221);
2. Extend the head and retest for tenderness;
3. Fine tune this position with slight head sidebending and rotation away from the tender point until tenderness is 2/10 or less;
4. Hold the position of relief for 90 seconds;
5. Slowly and passively return the head to neutral and retest for tenderness.

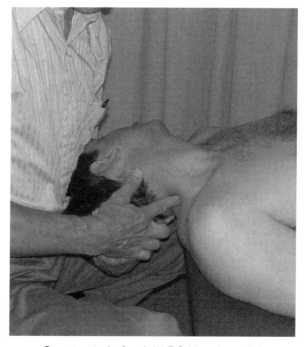

Counterstrain for right PC4 tender point

231

ANTERIOR C1 COUNTERSTRAIN

Indication: Tender point at C1 transverse process associated with neck pain, headache, and other problems.

Relative contraindications: Acute fracture or dislocation, atlantoaxial instability, vertebrobasilar insufficiency.

Technique (supine):

1. Locate the tender point at the C1 transverse process located between the angle of the mandible and the mastoid process, labeling it 10/10;
2. Rotate the head away from the tender point and retest for tenderness;
3. Fine tune this position with more rotation and slight flexion until tenderness is 2/10 or less;
4. Hold the position of relief for 90 seconds;
5. Slowly and passively return the head to neutral and retest for tenderness.

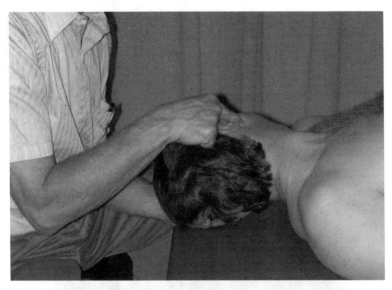

Right anterior C1 tender point and treatment position

ANTERIOR C2-C7 COUNTERSTRAIN

Indication: Anterior C2-C7 tender point associated with neck pain, headache, and other problems.

Relative contraindications: Acute cervical fracture or dislocation.

Technique (supine):

1. Locate the tender point on the anterior aspect of the articular pillar, labeling it 10/10 (see p.222);
2. Flex the head and retest for tenderness;
3. Fine tune this position with slight flexion, sidebending, and rotation until tenderness is 2/10 or less:
   AC2-C6 – usually sidebending and rotation away from tender point;
   AC7 – usually sidebending toward and rotation away from tender point;
4. Hold the position of relief for 90 seconds;
5. Slowly and passively return the head to neutral and retest for tenderness.

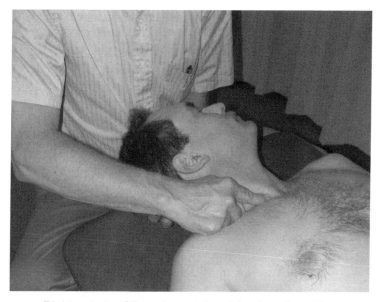

Right anterior C7 tender point and treatment position

CERVICAL MYOFASCIAL RELEASE

Indication: C2-C7 restriction related to neck pain, headache, and other problems.

Relative contraindications: Acute cervical fracture, vertebral cancer.

Technique (supine):

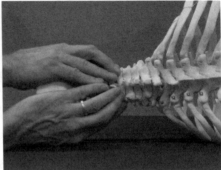

Hand position

1. Sitting at the head of the table, hold the occiput in your palms and place your fingertips at the lateral articular pillar on both sides of the restricted segment;
2. Indirect: Gently move the head and restricted segment to the position of sidebending, rotation, and flexion-extension laxity and follow any tissue release until completed;
3. Direct: Slowly move the head and restricted segment into the sidebending, rotation, and flexion-extension restrictions and apply steady force until tissue give is completed;
4. Retest sidebending.

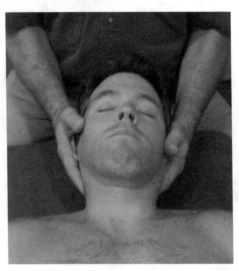

C3 myofascial release

CERVICAL LIGAMENTOUS ARTICULAR STRAIN

Indication: Cervical joint tension, tenderness, or restriction related to neck pain, headache, and other problems.

Relative contraindications: Acute cervical fracture, vertebral cancer.

Technique (supine):

1. Place your thenar eminences on the superior nuchal ridge medial to occipitomastoid sutures;
2. Place your fingertips on the articular pillars one segment below the somatic dysfunction;
3. Compress the somatic dysfunction by pushing your fingertips anteriorly and superiorly while pushing the occiput inferiorly;
4. Maintain compression until tissue give is completed;
5. Retest for joint somatic dysfunction.

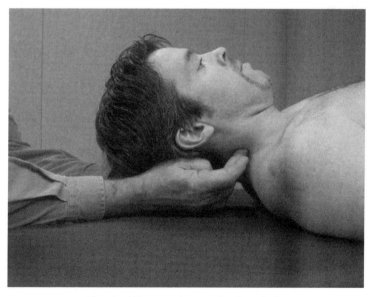

Cervical ligamentous articular strain

OCCIPITOATLANTAL MYOFASCIAL RELEASE

Indication: Restricted suboccipital fascia rotation related to neck pain, headache, upper respiratory congestion, and other problems.

Relative contraindications: Acute cervical fracture.

Technique (supine):

1. Place your fingertips on the skin in the suboccipital area and test fascial rotation right and left to identify restriction and laxity;
2. Indirect: Rotate the suboccipital fascia to its position of laxity and follow any tissue release until completed;
3. Direct: Rotate the suboccipital fascia into its restriction and apply steady force until tissue give is completed;
4. Retest suboccipital fascial rotation.

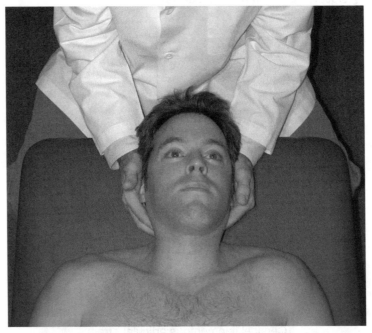

Occipitoatlantal myofascial release

CERVICAL SOFT TISSUE FACILITATED POSITIONAL RELEASE

Indications: Cervical paraspinal tension associated with neck pain, headache, and other problems.

Relative contraindications: Acute cervical fracture, vertebral cancer.

Technique (supine):

1. Sit at the head of the table and palpate the paraspinal tension with one hand;
2. Holding the top of the head with your other hand, slowly flex the neck to reduce the cervical lordosis;
3. Slowly sidebend and rotate the head toward the paraspinal tension until it decreases;
4. Slightly extend the head until paraspinal tension is further reduced;
5. Hold this position for 3–5 seconds until tension release is completed and slowly return the head to neutral;
6. Retest for paraspinal tension.

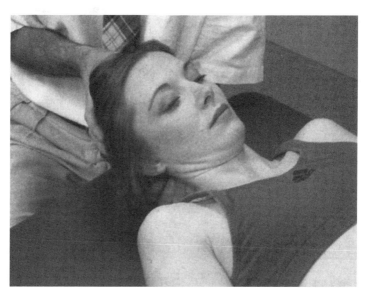

Cervical soft tissue FPR for right tension

SUBOCCIPITAL FACILITATED OSCILLATORY RELEASE

Indication: Suboccipital tension associated with neck pain, headache, and other problems.

Relative contraindications: Acute fracture, significant patient guarding.

Technique (supine):

1. Sit at the head of the table and gently hold the occiput in your palms;
2. Use one or two fingertips to apply focal pressure to tense tissues;
3. Move the head into flexion, rotation, or sidebending to apply positional stretch to the tense tissues;
4. While stabilizing the head, add gentle oscillatory motion through your finger contact by movement of the wrist in alternately opposite directions;
5. Continue oscillation until tension is reduced.

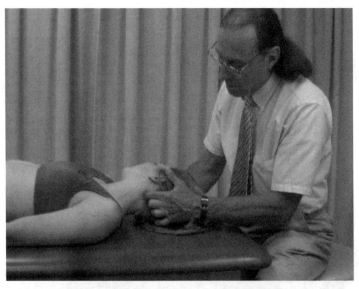

Suboccipital facilitated oscillatory release

CERVICAL SIDEBENDING MUSCLE ENERGY/THRUST

Indication: Restricted sidebending C2-C7 related to neck pain, headache, and other problems.

Relative contraindications: Joint inflammation, acute sprain, acute fracture, undiagnosed cervical radiculopathy, vertebral artery insufficiency, joint hypermobility (thrust only).

Technique (supine):

1. Hold the occiput in your palms and place your index finger at the superior aspect of the restricted segment with that arm pointing toward the opposite axilla;
2. Move the head into its flexion-extension and sidebending restrictive barriers around your MCP joint;
3. Rotate the head away from the sidebending restriction to better localize the barrier;
4. Ask the patient to sidebend the head away from the restriction into your equal resistance for 3–5 seconds;
5. Slowly move the head to a new sidebending restrictive barrier;
6. Repeat 3–5 times or until motion returns;
7. For thrust exert a short quick sidebending movement with your MCP joint toward the opposite axilla;
8. Retest cervical sidebending.

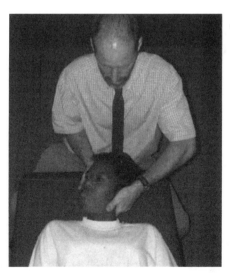

Sidebending muscle energy for C3 E RS right

239

CERVICAL ROTATION MUSCLE ENERGY/THRUST

Indication: Restricted rotation C2-C7 related to neck pain, headache, and other problems.

Relative contraindications: Joint inflammation, acute sprain, acute fracture, undiagnosed cervical radiculopathy, vertebral artery insufficiency, cervical joint hypermobility (thrust only).

Technique (supine):

1. Hold the occiput in your palms and place your index finger at the superior aspect of the restricted segment with that arm pointing toward the jaw;
2. Move the head into its flexion-extension and rotation restrictive barriers around your MCP joint;
3. Sidebend the head away from the rotation restriction to better localize the barrier;
4. Ask the patient to rotate the head away from the restriction into your equal resistance for 3–5 seconds;
5. Slowly move the head to a new rotation restrictive barrier;
6. Repeat 3–5 times or until motion returns;
7. For thrust exert a short quick rotational movement with your MCP joint toward the jaw;
8. Retest cervical rotation.

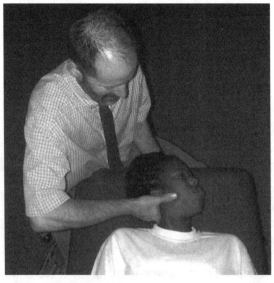

Rotational muscle energy for C3 F RS right

Indication: Restricted C2-C7 sidebending or rotation related to neck pain, headache, and other problems.

Relative contraindications: Joint inflammation, acute sprain, acute fracture, cervical joint hypermobility, undiagnosed cervical radiculopathy, vertebral cancer, vertebral artery insufficiency.

Technique:

1. Stand behind the patient and place your thumb on the inferior facet of the restricted segment to stabilize it;
2. Hold the forehead with your other hand and slowly induce neck movement into the rotation, sidebending, and flexion-extension positions of ease:
   a) Locked closed facet: Induce extension and sidebending-rotation toward it;
   b) Locked open facet: Induce flexion and sidebending-rotation away from it;
3. Slowly move the neck into the restrictive barrier for all planes and then slowly return to the positions of ease;
4. To facilitate return of motion, ask the patient to take a deep breath or to push the head away from the restriction for 3-5 seconds against your equal resistance, repeating as needed until motion returns;
5. Retest segmental sidebending or rotation.

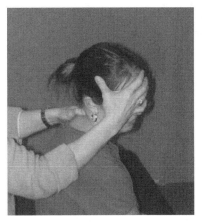 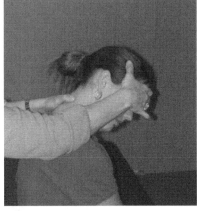

2a. C4 E RS right
(locked closed right)

2b. C4 F RS left
(locked open right)

CERVICAL SIDEBENDING ARTICULATORY – SUPINE

Indication: Restricted sidebending C2-C7 related to neck pain, headache, and other problems.

Relative contraindications: Joint inflammation, acute sprain, acute fracture, cervical joint hypermobility, undiagnosed cervical radiculopathy, vertebral cancer, vertebral artery insufficiency.

Technique:

1. Hold the patient's occiput in your palms;
2. Place your index finger at the superior aspect of the restricted segment and gently push toward the patient's opposite axilla;
3. In one smooth motion, slowly flex the head, sidebend it toward the restriction, rotate away from the restriction, and extend the head around your MCP joint;
4. Repeat 3–5 times or until joint mobility returns;
5. Retest cervical sidebending.

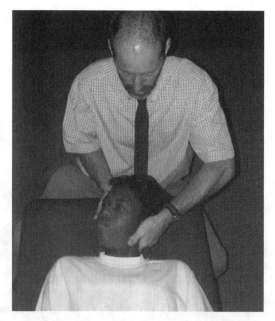

Sidebending articulatory for C3 RS right

CERVICAL ROTATION ARTICULATORY – SUPINE

Indication: Restricted rotation C2-C7 related to neck pain, headache, and other problems.

Relative contraindications: Joint inflammation, acute sprain, acute fracture, cervical joint hypermobility, undiagnosed cervical radiculopathy, vertebral cancer, vertebral artery insufficiency.

Technique:

1. Hold the patient's occiput in your palms;
2. Place your index finger at the superior aspect of the restricted segment and gently push toward the patient's jaw;
3. In one smooth motion, slowly flex the head, rotate it toward the restriction, sidebend away from the restriction, and extend the head around your MCP joint;
4. Repeat 3–5 times or until joint mobility occurs;
5. Retest cervical rotation.

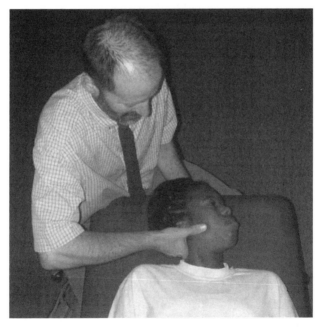

Rotation articulatory for C3 RS right

ATLANTOAXIAL MUSCLE ENERGY/THRUST

Indications: Restricted atlantoaxial (AA) rotation related to neck pain, headache, and other problems.

Relative contraindications: Acute fracture or dislocation, acute sprain, atlantoaxial instability, vertebrobasilar insufficiency.

Technique (supine):

1. Place your fingertips on the atlas in the suboccipital area and use your palms to gently lift the head to a flexion restrictive barrier;
2. Rotate the head and atlas right and left to identify a restriction, discontinuing if dizziness, nausea, diaphoresis, or nystagmus occurs;
3. Rotate the head and atlas to the rotation restrictive barrier and ask the patient to gently rotate the head away from the restriction against your equal resistance for 3-5 seconds;
4. Slowly move the head and atlas to a new rotation restrictive barrier;
5. Repeat 3-5 times or until motion returns;
6. For thrust, exert a short quick movement into the rotation restrictive barrier;
7. Retest atlantoaxial rotation.

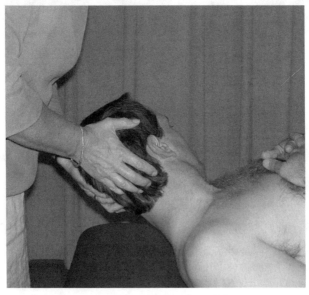

AA muscle energy for restricted left rotation

Indications: Restricted occipitoatlantal (OA) motion related to neck pain, headache, and other problems.

Relative contraindications: Acute fracture or dislocation, acute sprain, atlantoaxial instability, vertebrobasilar insufficiency.

Technique (supine):

1. Gently sidebend or translate the occiput in neutral, flexion, and extension to identify an occipitoatlantal restriction;
2. Discontinue if dizziness, nausea, diaphoresis, or nystagmus occurs;
3. Move the occiput into its flexion-extension and sidebending restrictive barriers and ask the patient to gently sidebend the head away from the restriction against your equal resistance for 3-5 seconds;
4. Slowly move the head to a new sidebending restrictive barrier;
5. Repeat 3-5 times or until motion returns;
6. For thrust, apply a short quick movement into the sidebending or rotation restrictive barrier;
7. Retest occipitoatlantal motion.

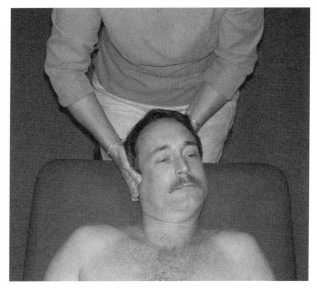

Muscle energy for OA E S left R right

POSTERIOR CERVICAL POSITION OF EASE

1. Lying on your back, insert a small pillow or rolled up towel behind your neck;
2. Allow your head to drop back over the pillow and rest on the floor;
3. If comfortable, take a few deep breaths and rest in this position for 2-5 minutes if no dizziness, blurred vision, or nausea occurs;
4. Remove the pillow and roll to one side before slowly getting up;
5. Use this position 2-4 times a day or as needed for pain relief.

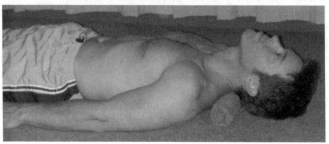

Posterior cervical position of ease

CERVICAL EXTENSOR STRETCH

1. Sit with your feet flat on the floor;
2. Place your hands on the back of the head;
3. Keeping the back straight, let the chin drop down toward the chest and allow the weight of your arms to pull the head down;
4. Take a few deep breaths and stretch for 10-20 seconds;
5. Do this stretch 1-4 times a day.

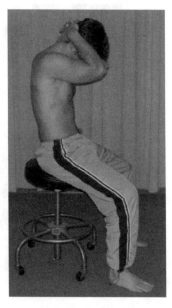

Cervical extensor stretch

TRAPEZIUS STRETCH

1. While sitting, hold on to the chair with one hand;
2. Hold the top of your head with the other hand;
3. Allow the head to slowly fall to the side away from the tight trapezius muscle as far as it will comfortably go, letting the weight of the arm move the head;
4. Take a few deep breaths and stretch for 10-20 seconds;
5. Repeat to the other side;
6. Do this stretch 1-4 times a day.

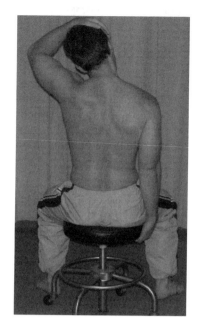

Trapezius stretch

LEVATOR STRETCH

1. While seated, hold onto the chair with one hand;
2. Hold the top of your head with the other hand with fingertips just above the opposite ear;
3. Allow the head to slowly fall first forward and then to the side away from the tight levator scapula muscle as far as it will comfortably go;
4. Take a few deep breaths and stretch for 10-20 seconds;
5. Repeat for the other side;
6. Do this stretch 1-4 times a day.

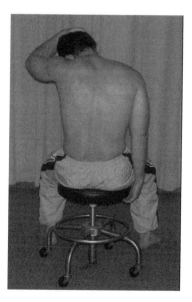

Levator stretch

SCALENE POSITION OF EASE

1. Lie on your back with the head resting on one or two pillows;
2. Bend the head to the side of neck pain;
3. If comfortable, take a few deep breaths and rest in this position for 2-5 minutes;
4. Slowly roll to one side before getting up;
5. Repeat 2-4 times a day or as needed for pain relief.

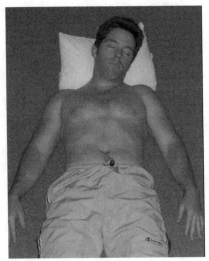

Scalene position of ease

SCALENE STRETCH

1. While seated, hold onto the chair with one hand;
2. Hold the top of the head with your other hand;
3. Allow the head to slowly fall to the side away from the tight scalene muscles as far as it will comfortably go, letting the weight of arm move the head;
4. Take a few deep breaths and stretch for 10-20 seconds;
5. Repeat steps 3-4 with the head bent slightly backward;
6. Repeat these stretches for the other side;
7. Do this stretch 1-4 times a day.

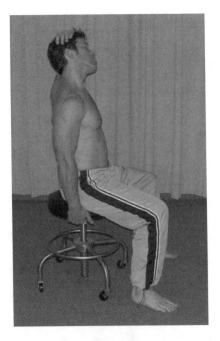

Scalene stretch

STERNOCLEIDOMASTOID (SCM) POSITION OF EASE

1. Lie on your back with the head resting on one or two pillows;
2. With the head bent slightly toward the side of neck pain, allow the head to rotate away from the side of pain;
3. If comfortable, take a few deep breaths and rest in this position for 2-5 minutes;
4. Slowly roll to one side before getting up;
5. Repeat 2-4 times a day or as needed for pain relief.

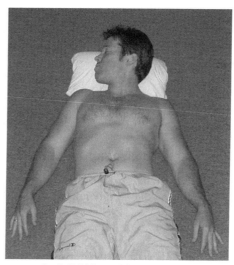

Left SCM position of ease

STERNOCLEIDOMASTOID STRETCH

1. Lie on your back with the head resting on a pillow;
2. Allow the head to turn to one side as far as is comfortable;
3. With one hand on the cheek, allow the weight of the arm to turn the head farther;
4. Take a few deep breaths and stretch for 10-20 seconds, stopping sooner if there is dizziness, blurred vision, or nausea;
5. Repeat to the other side;
6. Do this stretch 1-4 times a day.

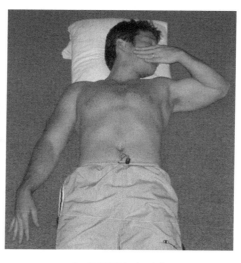

Left SCM stretch

CERVICAL JOINT POSITION OF EASE

1. Lying on your back, insert a small pillow or rolled up towel under the neck;
2. Allow the head to fall back around the pillow;
3. Slowly turn the head away from the side of neck pain until it decreases;
4. If comfortable, take a few deep breaths and rest in this position for 2-5 minutes unless dizziness, blurred vision, or nausea develop;
5. Slowly remove the pillow and roll to one side before getting up;
6. Use this position 2-4 times a day or as needed for pain relief.

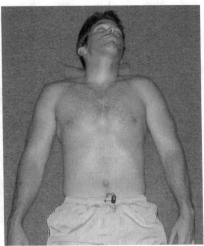

Cervical joint position of ease

CERVICAL SIDEBENDING MOBILIZATION

1. Lie on your back and use one hand to grip both sides of the back of the neck just below the restricted area;
2. Use the other hand to gently and repetitively move the head into sidebending around the hand at the back of the neck;
3. Repeat for the other side if needed;
4. Do up to twice a day if helpful.

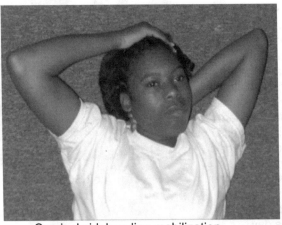

Cervical sidebending mobilization

REFERENCE

1. AMA. *Guides to the Evaluation of Permanent Impairment, 4th Edition.* American Medical Association, Chicago, 1994.

CERVICAL NOTES

CERVICAL NOTES (cont.)

Chapter 10: CRANIAL DIAGNOSIS AND TREATMENT

Diagnosis of Cranial Somatic Dysfunction

1. Screening
    a) Cranial palpation – p.258
    b) Cranial motion testing – p.259
        Vault hold – p.259
        Fronto-occipital hold – p.260
        Posterior temporal hold – p.260
2. Temporomandibular joint (TMJ) palpation/motion testing – p.261
3. Cranial somatic dysfunction – pp.262-263
4. Neurological exam before treatment
    a) Cranial nerve exam if indicated
    b) Funduscopic exam if indicated
    c) Extremity neurological exam if indicated

Treatment of Cranial Somatic Dysfunction

1. OMT

Facial effleurage – p.264
Venous sinus drainage – pp.265-266
Compression of the 4th ventricle – p.267
Frontal lift – p.268
Parietal lift – p.269
SBS compression-decompression – p.270
Trigeminal stimulation – p.271
Sphenopalatine ganglion stimulation – p.272
Temporal decompression – p.273
TMJ compression/decompression – p.274
V-spread (suture disengagement) – p.275
Mandibular drainage – p.276
Occipital decompression – p.277
Balanced membranous tension – p.278

2. Exercises

Cervical extensor stretch – see p.246
Trigeminal stimulation – p.279
TMJ mobilization – p.280

3. Thermal therapy

Heat 20-30 minutes 4-6 times a day for tension or stiffness
Cold 15-20 minutes 4-6 times a day for pain relief

4. Stabilization

TMJ orthotic if bite asymmetry

CRANIAL PALPATION

1. Palpate the following cranial sutures for tenderness:

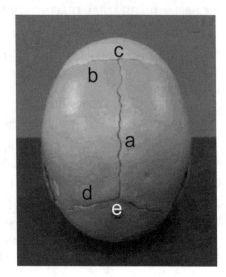
Superior cranial landmarks

a) Sagittal suture – midline between parietal bones;
b) Coronal suture – between parietal and frontal bones;
c) Bregma – juncture of sagittal and coronal sutures;
d) Lambdoidal suture – between parietal bones and occiput;
e) Lambda – juncture of sagittal and lambdoidal sutures;
f) Occipitomastoid suture – between occiput and mastoid processes;
g) Asterion – juncture of occiput, parietal, and temporal bones;
h) Squamosal suture – between parietal and temporal bones;
i) Pterion – juncture of frontal, parietal, sphenoid, and temporal bones;
j) Metopic suture – midline between two halves of frontal bone in children and some adults (not shown).

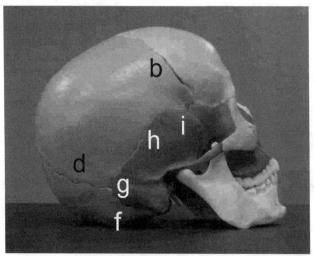
Lateral cranial landmarks

CRANIAL MOTION TESTING

1. Using the hold of your choice, palpate the following unpaired midline cranial bones for flexion and extension:

    a) Occiput
    b) Sphenoid
    c) Mandible

2. Using the hold of your choice, palpate the following paired cranial bones for external and internal rotation:

    a) Parietal
    b) Frontal
    c) Temporal
    d) Zygoma
    e) Maxilla
    f) Nasal

VAULT HOLD

1. Gently hold the sides of the head with index fingers on sphenoid greater wings, third and fourth fingertips anterior and posterior to the ears, and fifth fingertips on the occipital bone;
2. Your thumbs are resting lightly on the vertex of the head;
3. Follow the cranial rhythmic impulse and evaluate for rate, amplitude, and symmetry.

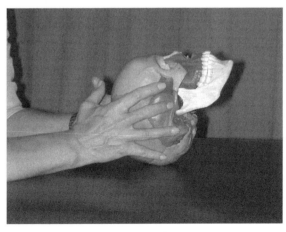

Vault hold

FRONTO-OCCIPITAL HOLD

1. Let the occiput rest in one hand, avoiding pressure on the occipitomastoid sutures;
2. Let your other hand rest on the frontal bone just above the eyebrows with the thumb on one greater wing of sphenoid and middle fingertip on the other greater wing;
3. Follow the cranial rhythmic impulse and evaluate for rate, amplitude, and symmetry.

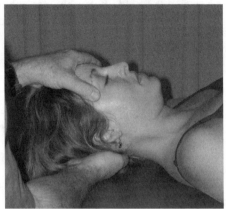

Fronto-occipital hold

POSTERIOR TEMPORAL HOLD

1. Gently hold the temporal bones with your thumbs on the sphenoid greater wings, index fingers posterior to the ears, and fifth fingertips on the squamous portion of the occipital bone;
2. Follow the cranial rhythmic impulse and evaluate for rate, amplitude, and symmetry.

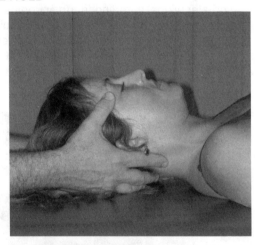

Posterior temporal hold

260

TEMPOROMANDIBULAR PALPATION/MOTION TESTING

1. Place your first and second fingertips at the temporomandibular (TMJ) joints located just anterior to the lower earlobes;
2. Palpate for tenderness and asymmetry;
3. Ask the patient to slowly open the mouth as far as possible;
4. The mandible normally opens symmetrically without crepitus in the joints;
5. Deviation of the mandible to one side during opening indicates TMJ restriction on that side.

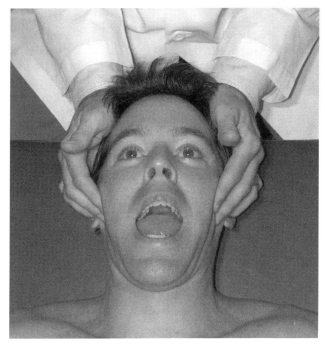

TMJ palpation and motion testing

CRANIAL SOMATIC DYSFUNCTION

Somatic Dysfunction	Exam Findings	Etiology
Slow rate	CRI[1] rate < 10 cycles/minute	Slow metabolism Chronic infection Chronic fatigue
Fast rate	CRI rate > 14 cycles/minute	Fast metabolism Acute infection
Low amplitude	CRI amplitude < 3/5	Dural tension SBS[2] compression
SBS[2] torsion	Sphenoid and occiput rotate in opposite direction around an A-P axis	Postural strain Cervical dysfunction Head trauma May be normal
SBS[2] sidebending rotation	Sphenoid and occiput rotate in same direction around an A-P axis and in opposite direction around parallel vertical axes	Postural strain Cervical somatic dysfunction Head trauma May be normal
SBS[2] vertical strain	Sphenoid and occiput rotate in same direction around parallel transverse axes	Head trauma
SBS[2] lateral strain	Sphenoid and occiput rotate in same direction around parallel vertical axes	Head trauma
SBS[2] compression	Sphenoid and occiput have little or no mobility	Head trauma Depression Severe emotional trauma
Internal rotation	Paired bone restricted in external rotation	Head trauma Dural tension
External rotation	Paired bone restricted in internal rotation	Head trauma Dural tension
TMJ dysfunction	TMJ tenderness, crepitus, and restricted opening	Myofascial strain Dental malocclusion Cranial dysfunction Joint degeneration

[1]Cranial rhythmic impulse normals: Rate = 10-14 cycles per minute; Amplitude = 3-5/5; Rhythm = symmetrical.
[2]Sphenobasilar synchondrosis at juncture of sphenoid and occiput.

Somatic Dysfunction	Right Sphenoid Greater Wing	Left Sphenoid Greater Wing	Right Occiput	Left Occiput
Right torsion[1]	superior	inferior	inferior	superior
Left torsion[1]	inferior	superior	superior	inferior
Right sidebending rotation[2]	inferior and anterior	superior and posterior	inferior and posterior	superior and anterior
Left sidebending rotation[2]	superior and posterior	inferior and anterior	superior and anterior	inferior and posterior
Right lateral strain[3]	medial and anterior	lateral and posterior	lateral and anterior	medial and posterior
Left lateral strain[3]	lateral and posterior	medial and anterior	medial and posterior	lateral and anterior
Inferior vertical strain[3]	superior	superior	inferior	inferior
Superior vertical strain[3]	inferior	inferior	superior	superior
Compression	no motion	no motion	no motion	no motion

[1]Torsions are named for the superior greater wing of the sphenoid.
[2]Sidebending rotations are named for the side of head convexity.
[3]Sphenobasilar strains are named for the direction of basisphenoid movement which is opposite to greater wing movement.

FACIAL EFFLEURAGE

Indications: Tension headache, upper respiratory congestion, and other problems.

Relative contraindications: Intracranial bleed, craniofacial fracture, CNS malignancy or infection, cystic acne.

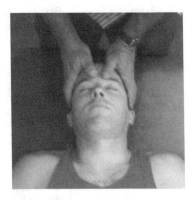

Step 1: Frontal

Technique (seated or supine):

1. Place your thumbs at the midline of the forehead and firmly slide them laterally over the skin toward the ears;
2. Place your thumbs at the bridge of the nose and firmly slide them laterally over the skin toward the angles of the mandible;
3. Place your thumbs at the midline of the mandible and firmly slide them laterally over the skin toward the angles of the mandible;
4. Place your fingertips inferior to the ears and firmly slide them inferiorly over the skin toward the medial clavicles, avoiding pressure on the carotid arteries;
5. Repeat each step as often as needed to facilitate drainage.

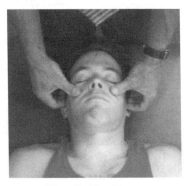

Step 2: Maxilla

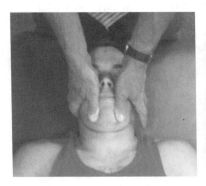

Step 3: Mandible

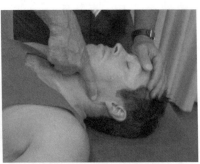

Step 4: Lateral neck

VENOUS SINUS DRAINAGE

Indications: Headache, upper respiratory congestion, and other problems.

Relative contraindications: Intracranial bleed, craniofacial fracture, CNS malignancy or infection.

Technique (supine):

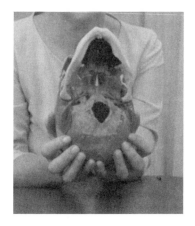

1. Seated at the head of the table, align your fingertips along the superior nuchal ridge with fifth fingers on the inion and exert slight anterior and lateral pressure until tissue give is completed;
2. Align your fingertips on both sides of the midline of the occipital bone with fifth fingers on the inion and exert slight superior and lateral pressure until tissue give is completed;

Step 1: Transverse sinus

3. Cross your thumbs and contact the opposite parietal bone on both sides of the sagittal suture at lambda, exerting slight inferior and lateral pressure until tissue give is completed and repeating anteriorly along the sagittal suture until reaching bregma;
4. Align your fingertips on both sides of the metopic suture or along the midline of the frontal bone and exert slight posterior and lateral pressure until tissue give is completed.

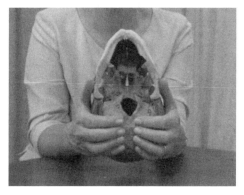

Step 2: Occipital sinus

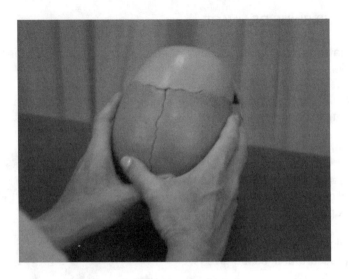

Step 3: Superior sagittal sinus

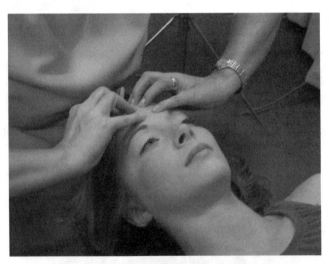

Step 4: Superior sagittal sinus at metopic suture

COMPRESSION OF THE 4ᵗᴴ VENTRICLE (CV4)

Indication: Diminished cranial rhythmic impulse (CRI) amplitude related to headache, upper respiratory congestion, and other problems.

Relative contraindications: Intracranial bleed, craniofacial fracture, CNS malignancy or infection.

Technique (supine):

1. Sit at the head of the table and place one hand on top of the other with the thenar eminences aligned;
2. Place the thenar eminences on the occipital bone inferior to the superior nuchal ridge and medial to the occipitomastoid sutures;
3. Palpate cranial flexion and extension and use your hands and intention to gently encourage extension and resist flexion until the CRI stops at a still point;
4. Maintain this extension still point until CRI flexion returns and then gently release pressure to allow full flexion. If unable to feel the CRI, allow the occiput to rest on your hands for 1-2 minutes without exerting pressure;
5. Reexamine CRI amplitude.

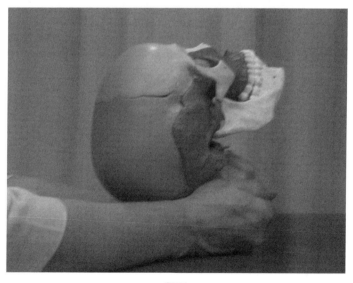

CV4

FRONTAL LIFT

Indications: Restricted frontal mobility associated with headache, depression, sinus congestion, pediatric development abnormalities, and other problems.

Relative contraindications: Intracranial bleed, craniofacial fracture, CNS malignancy or infection.

Technique (supine):

1. Sit at the head of the table and use your fingertips to gently contact the frontal bone posterior to the orbital ridge on both sides;
2. Palpate the cranial rhythmic impulse or gently apply anterior traction to identify restricted frontal mobility;
3. Gently lift the frontal bone anteriorly until slight give is equal on both sides;
4. Reexamine frontal mobility.

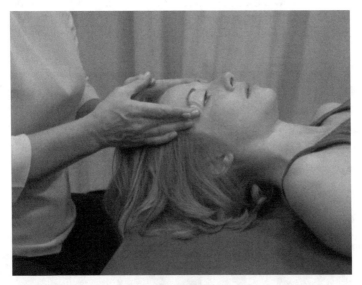

Frontal lift

PARIETAL LIFT

Indications: Restricted parietal mobility associated with headache, upper respiratory congestion, pediatric development abnormalities, and other problems.

Relative contraindications: Intracranial bleed, craniofacial fracture, CNS malignancy or infection.

Technique (supine):

1. Sit at the head of the table and use your fingertips to gently contact the lateral aspect of the parietal bones superior to the squamous sutures, with your thumbs crossed but off the top of the head;
2. Palpate the cranial rhythmic impulse to identify restricted parietal mobility;
3. Gently press medially into the parietal bones until slight give is equal on both sides;
4. Gently lift the parietal bones superiorly until slight give is equal on both sides;
5. Reexamine parietal mobility.

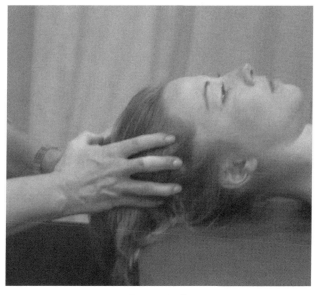

Parietal lift

SBS COMPRESSION-DECOMPRESSION

Indication: Diminished CRI amplitude (SBS compression) related to headache, mood disorders, cranial nerve entrapment, upper respiratory congestion, pediatric development abnormalities, and other problems.

Relative contraindications: Intracranial bleed, craniofacial fracture, CNS malignancy or infection.

Technique (supine):

1. Using the posterior temporal or fronto-occipital hold, gently compress the SBS by moving the sphenoid greater wings posteroinferiorly and the occiput anterosuperiorly until slight give is equal on both sides;
2. Gently decompress the SBS by lifting the sphenoid greater wings anterosuperiorly until slight give is equal on both sides;
3. Slowly release decompression and reexamine the CRI for return of sphenoid and occiput mobility.

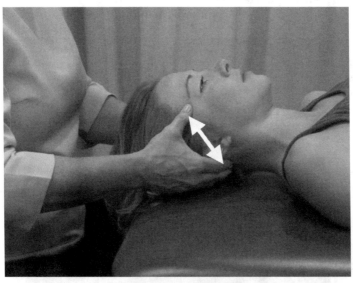

SBS decompression

TRIGEMINAL STIMULATION

Indications: Tenderness at the trigeminal foramina associated with upper respiratory congestion and other problems.

Relative contraindications: Intracranial bleed, craniofacial fracture, CNS malignancy or infection.

Technique (supine, seated, standing):

1. Use a finger to palpate trigeminal foramina which can be identified as a small depression at the following locations:
    Ophthalmic division (VI) – supraorbital notch on the medial supraorbital ridge;
    Maxillary division (V2) – infraorbital foramen on the medial infraorbital ridge;
    Mandibular division (V3) – mental foramen on the anterior body of the mandible;
2. Press directly into a tender trigeminal foramen with or without rotatory pressure for 10 seconds.

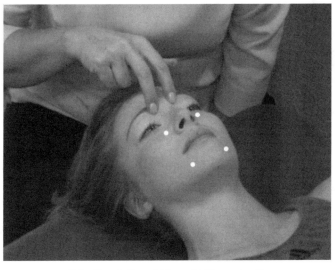

V1 stimulation (V2 and V3 marked)

SPHENOPALATINE GANGLION STIMULATION

Indications: Upper respiratory congestion and other problems.

Relative contraindications: Intracranial bleed, craniofacial fracture, CNS malignancy or infection.

Technique (supine):

1. Stand on the opposite side and insert the gloved fifth digit of your caudad hand into the mouth and along the outside of the upper molars, palpating posteriorly and then superiorly until you feel a small depression at the back roof of the mouth;
2. Exert slight pressure into this depression until tender or have the patient nod into your finger to tolerance for 3 seconds;
3. Repeat 3-5 times or until the eye starts tearing on that side;
4. Repeat on the other side if needed.

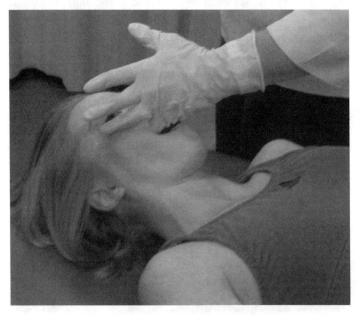

Sphenopalatine ganglion stimulation

TEMPORAL DECOMPRESSION

Indications: Restricted temporal mobility associated with headache, otitis media, vertigo, tinnitus, TMJ syndrome, and other problems.

Relative contraindications: Intracranial bleed, craniofacial fracture, CNS malignancy or infection.

Technique (supine):

1. Sit at the head of the table and gently grasp the posterior earlobes between your thumbs and fingertips;
2. Gently pull the ears in a posterolateral direction until slight give is equal on both sides;
3. Reexamine temporal mobility.

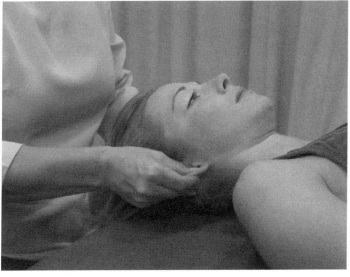

Temporal decompression

TMJ COMPRESSION/DECOMPRESSION

Indication: Temporomandibular joint (TMJ) restriction related to TMJ pain, mandible restriction, neck pain, and other problems.

Relative contraindications: Craniofacial fracture.

Technique (supine):

1. Sit at the head of the table and place your fingertips under the body of the mandible;
2. Gently pull the mandible superiorly toward the TMJ until slight give is equal on both sides;
3. Move your fingertips to the lateral mandible and gently push it inferiorly away from the TMJ until slight give is equal on both sides;
4. Retest TMJ mobility.

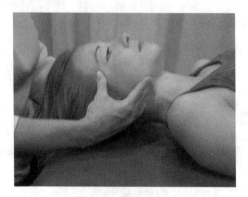

TMJ compression

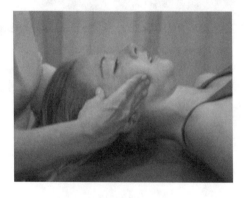

TMJ decompression

V-SPREAD (suture disengagement)

Indications: Suture tenderness or cranial bone restriction associated with headache, cranial nerve entrapment, and other problems.

Relative contraindications: Intracranial bleed, craniofacial fracture, CNS malignancy or infection.

Technique (supine):

1. Contact the bone on either side of the suture with your index and middle finger of one hand and apply steady traction to separate the suture;
2. Place the index and middle finger of your other hand on the opposite side of the head and exert a slight repetitive impulse toward the restricted suture;
3. Continue sutural traction and contralateral impulse until sutural give is finished;
4. Retest cranial bone mobility.

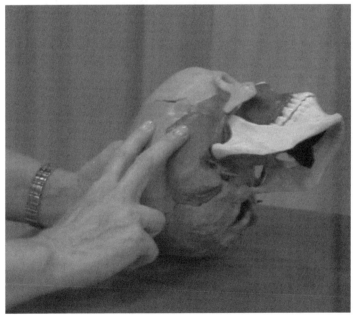

Squamous suture disengagement

MANDIBULAR DRAINAGE (Galbreath)

Indications: Otitis media, eustachian insufficiency, and other problems.

Relative contraindications: Intracranial bleed, craniofacial fracture, CNS malignancy or infection, temporomandibular joint subluxation.

Technique (supine):

1. Standing at one side of the head, gently hold the forehead and rotate the head toward you so the opposite eustachian tube is positioned with a downward slant toward the oropharynx;
2. Hold the angle of the opposite mandible with your fingertips;
3. Gently pull the mandible anteriorly until slight tension is encountered and then release, repeating this pull and release rhythmically for one minute;
4. Repeat for the other side if needed.

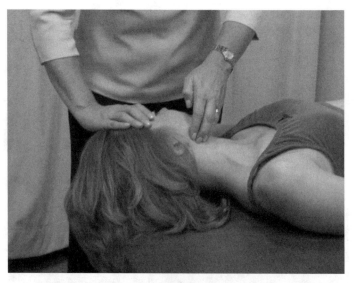

Mandibular drainage for the right eustachian tube

OCCIPITAL DECOMPRESSION

Indications: Restricted occipital mobility associated with infant feeding disorders, colic, congenital muscular torticollis, and other problems.

Relative contraindications: Intracranial bleed, craniofacial fracture, CNS malignancy or infection.

Technique (supine):

1. Sit at the head of the infant and gently contact the cranial base with index fingers on mastoid processes, middle fingers on occipital condyles, and ring fingers on supraocciput;
2. Gently pull the occiput in a posterior, then lateral direction while resisting mastoid process movement until slight occipital give is completed equally on both sides;
3. Reexamine occipital mobility.

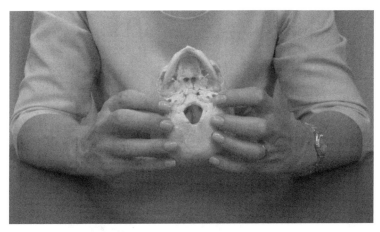

Hand placement for occipital decompression

BALANCED MEMBRANOUS TENSION

Indication: Asymmetrical or diminished cranial rhythmic impulse (CRI) related to headache, cranial nerve entrapment, and other problems.

Relative contraindications: Intracranial bleed, craniofacial fracture, CNS malignancy or infection.

Technique (supine):

1. Use the vault hold to palpate the CRI to identify asymmetry of motion secondary to intracranial membranous strain;
2. Indirect: Gently use your hands and intention to exaggerate membranous asymmetry;
3. Continue exaggerating membranous asymmetry and resisting return to neutral until the CRI stops at a still point;
4. Maintain this position until the CRI returns and then gently follow it back to neutral before releasing pressure;
5. Reexamine the CRI and membranes for return of symmetry.

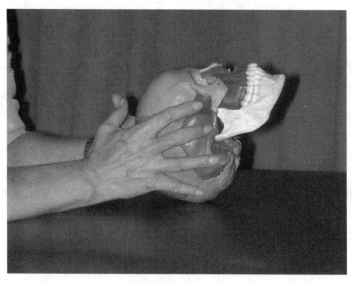

Hand position for balanced membranous tension

1. Slide your fingertip outward along the eyebrow until you contact a tender depression in the bone;
2. Exert rotatory pressure at this depression for 10 seconds;
3. Place your fingertip at the top of the nose and slide it down along the face beside the nose until you contact a tender depression;
4. Exert rotatory pressure at this depression for 10 seconds;
5. Repeat for one or both sides as often as needed to relieve nasal congestion.

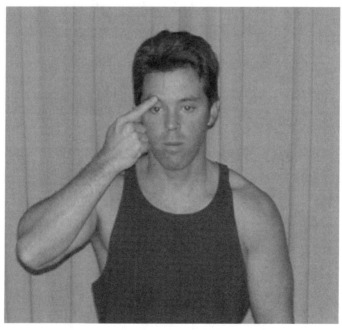

Trigeminal stimulation at supraorbital notch

TMJ MOBILIZATION[1]

1. Place the back of the knuckles of one or two fingers between upper and lower teeth;
2. Gently bite down into the fingers for 5-15 seconds;
3. Repeat 2-3 times if needed;
4. Do this exercise 2-4 times a day if helpful.

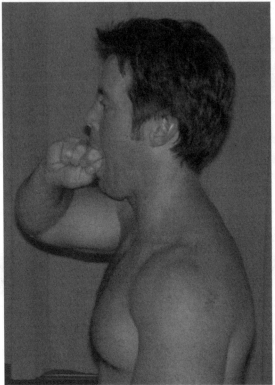

TMJ mobilization

REFERENCE

1. Folio LR. *A new osteopathic manipulative technique in home-care management of temporomandibular joint pain.* Student Doctor January/February 1986:8-11. 1986.

UPPER EXTREMITY NOTES

Diagnosis of Upper Extremity Somatic Dysfunction
1. Screening
    a) Arm abduction – p.286
    b) Shoulder palpation – pp.287-288
2. Motion testing – integrated into OMT and:
    a) Glenohumeral abduction – p.295, p.297
    b) Sternoclavicular motion – p.301
    c) Elbow/forearm exam – p.305
3. Upper extremity somatic dysfunction – p.291
4. Neurological exam if indicated:
    a) Upper extremity deep tendon reflexes, strength, sensation
    b) Thoracic outlet syndrome exam – pp.289-290
    c) Carpal tunnel syndrome exam
5. Orthopedic exam if indicated

Treatment of Upper Extremity Somatic Dysfunction
1. OMT
Supraspinatus counterstrain – p.292
Acromioclavicular counterstrain – p.293
Scapula myofascial release – p.294
Glenohumeral myofascial release – p.296
Shoulder muscle energy – pp.297-299
Glenohumeral articulatory – p.300
Sternoclavicular muscle energy – pp.302-303
Sternoclavicular thrust – p.304
Elbow myofascial release – p.306
Elbow percussion vibrator – p.307
Ulna articulatory – p.308

Radial head counterstrain – p.309
Radial head thrust – p.310
Interosseous membrane soft tissue release – p.311
Forearm muscle energy – p.312
Wrist myofascial release – p.313
Carpal tunnel myofascial release – p.314
Wrist articulatory – p.315
Carpal articulatory – p.316
Upper extremity facilitated oscillatory release – p.317
Thumb metacarpal thrust – p.318
Interphalangeal articulatory – p.319

2. Exercises
Scalene position of ease – see p.248
Scalene stretch – see p.248
Rib 1mobilization – see p.212
Pectoral stretch – see p.211
Shoulder abductor position of ease – p.320
Shoulder abductor stretch – p.321

Shoulder mobilization – p.321
Wrist extensor position of ease – p.322
Wrist extensor stretch – p.322
Radial head mobilization – p.323
Carpal tunnel stretch – p.324

3. Thermal therapy
Heat 20-30 minutes 4-6 times a day for tension or stiffness
Cold 15-20 minutes 4-6 times a day for pain relief or inflammation

4. Stabilization
Brace for joint instability, lateral epicondylitis
Splint for carpal tunnel syndrome
Prolotherapy for ligament laxity

ARM ABDUCTION SCREENING

1. Have the standing patient slowly abduct both arms as far as possible, keeping the palms turned outward as the hands reach above the head;
2. Observe symmetry and amount of abduction (normal = 180°). Common causes of restricted abduction: shoulder problems, elbow problems, forearm problems;
3. Observe inferior angle of scapula rotation relative to shoulder abduction (normal scapulohumeral rhythm = 1° scapula rotation for every 2° humeral abduction). Decreased scapula rotation = shoulder girdle problem. Decreased humeral abduction = shoulder joint problem.

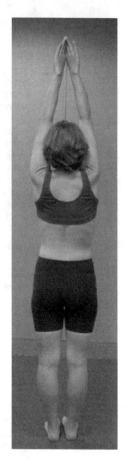

Arm abduction 180°

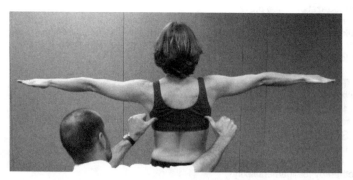

Scapulohumeral rhythm

1. With the patient seated or supine, palpate the following structures for tenderness:

   1) Sternoclavicular joint;
   2) Coracoid process – inferior to lateral clavicle, pectoralis minor insertion;
   3) Acromioclavicular joint;
      Subacromial bursa anterior and inferior to acromion with shoulder extension;
   4) Greater tuberosity of humerus – inferior to acromion, supraspinatus insertion;
   5) Lesser tuberosity of humerus – medial to greater tuberosity, subscapularis insertion;
      Bicipital groove between greater and lesser tuberosity;
   6) Glenohumeral joint line;
   7) Deltoid bursa.

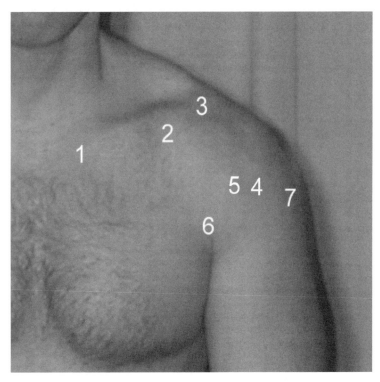

Locations of anterior shoulder tenderness

SHOULDER PALPATION – POSTERIOR

1. With the patient seated or prone, palpate the following structures for tenderness or tension:

    1) Levator scapula muscle;
    2) Upper trapezius muscle;
    3) Supraspinatus muscle;
    4) Infraspinatus muscle;
    5) Posterior axillary fold – teres minor, subscapularis, latissimus dorsi muscles;
    6) Rhomboid muscle;
    7) Glenohumeral joint line.

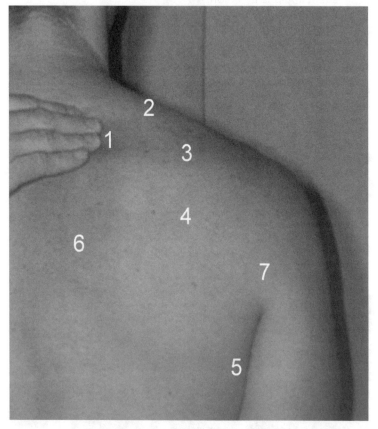

Locations of posterior shoulder tenderness

COSTOCLAVICULAR COMPRESSION TEST

Indication: Arm pain, numbness, or tingling.

1. Hold the wrist of the involved arm and palpate the radial pulse;
2. Ask the patient to sit up straight and use your hand and body weight to slowly push the clavicle posteroinferiorly;
3. Diminished pulse and reproduction or exacerbation of arm pain, numbness, or tingling indicate probable thoracic outlet syndrome from compression of the brachial plexus between clavicle and first rib.

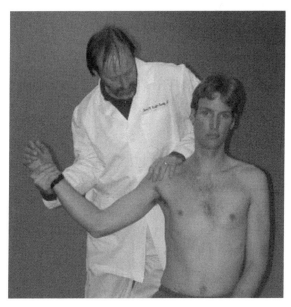

Costoclavicular compression test

PECTORALIS MINOR COMPRESSION TEST

Indication: Arm pain, numbness, or tingling.

1. With the patient seated or supine, palpate the radial pulse;
2. Passively extend and abduct the shoulder to its motion barrier to stretch the pectoralis minor muscle;
3. Diminished pulse and reproduction or exacerbation of arm pain, numbness, or tingling indicate probable thoracic outlet syndrome from pectoralis minor tendon compression of the brachial plexus.

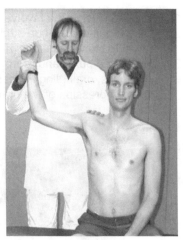

Pectoralis compression test

SCALENE COMPRESSION TEST (Adson maneuver)

Indication: Arm pain, numbness, or tingling.

1. Palpate the radial pulse, ask the patient to take a deep breath and hold it, and bend the head backward and rotate toward the side of the radial pulse being tested;
2. Diminished pulse and reproduction or exacerbation of arm pain, numbness, or tingling indicate probable thoracic outlet syndrome from compression of the brachial plexus between anterior and middle scalene muscles.

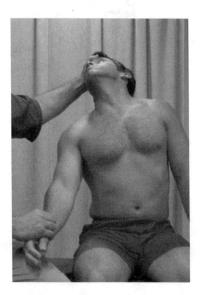

Scalene compression test

290

Somatic Dysfunction (position of laxity)	Diagnostic Finding
Tender points	Tender point at described location
Scapula	Restricted superior, inferior, medial, lateral, or rotation glide
Glenohumeral adduction, abduction, flexion, extension, internal rotation, external rotation	Restricted opposite motion
Clavicle superior	Restricted inferior glide at sternoclavicular (SC) joint with upward shoulder shrug
Clavicle inferior	Restricted superior glide at SC joint with downward shoulder shrug
Clavicle anterior	Restricted posterior glide at SC joint with forward shoulder shrug
Ulna abduction	Restricted adduction (lateral glide) at humeroulnar joint
Ulna adduction	Restricted abduction (medial glide) at humeroulnar joint
Forearm supination, pronation	Restricted opposite motion
Radial head posterior	Restricted anterior glide with supination
Radial head anterior	Restricted posterior glide with pronation
Wrist abduction, adduction, flexion, extension	Restricted opposite motion
Metacarpal flexion, extension, abduction, adduction	Restricted opposite motion
Interphalangeal flexion, extension, abduction, adduction	Restricted opposite motion

SUPRASPINATUS COUNTERSTRAIN

Indication: Tender point in supraspinatus muscle or tendon associated with shoulder pain, arm pain, back pain, and other problems.

Relative contraindications: Acute shoulder fracture or dislocation.

Technique (supine or lateral):

1. Locate the tender point in the supraspinatus muscle or its insertion onto the greater tuberosity of the humerus, labeling it 10/10;
2. Use your other hand to slowly abduct the arm about 45° and retest for tenderness;
3. Fine tune this position with slight arm external rotation until tenderness is 2/10 or less;
4. Hold the position of relief for 90 seconds;
5. Slowly and passively return the arm to neutral and retest for tenderness.

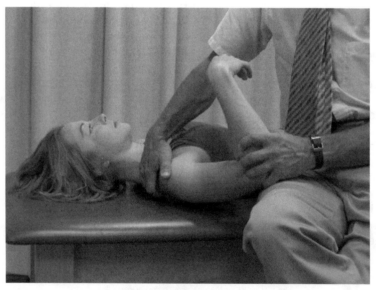

Supraspinatus counterstrain

ACROMIOCLAVICULAR COUNTERSTRAIN

Indication: Tender point at the acromioclavicular joint associated with shoulder pain, arm pain, and other problems.

Relative contraindications: Acute shoulder sprain, dislocation, or fracture.

Technique (supine):

1. Locate the tender point at the anterior acromioclavicular joint, labeling it 10/10;
2. Hold the wrist, flex and adduct the shoulder, and apply slight traction down the arm;
3. Retest for tenderness;
4. Fine tune this position with slight changes in adduction and traction until tenderness is 2/10 or less;
5. Hold the position of relief for 90 seconds;
6. Slowly and passively return the arm to neutral and retest for tenderness.

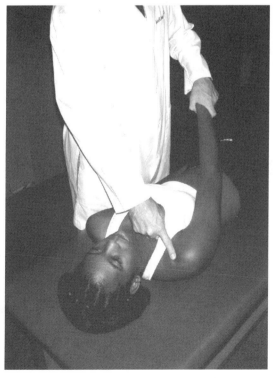

Acromioclavicular counterstrain

SCAPULA MYOFASCIAL RELEASE

Indication: Scapula restriction or tension related to shoulder pain, arm pain, back pain, chest wall pain, and other problems.

Relative contraindications: Acute scapula fracture.

Technique (lateral):

1. Stand facing the patient and drape the involved arm over your caudad hand which is holding the inferior angle of the scapula;
2. Hold the acromion and superior scapula with your other hand;
3. Slowly move the scapula into superior and inferior glide, medial and lateral glide, and lateral and medial rotation, determining directions of laxity and restriction;
4. Indirect: Slowly move the scapula into its positions of laxity and follow any tissue release until completed;
5. Direct: Slowly move the scapula into its restrictions and apply steady force until tissue give is completed;
6. Slowly return to neutral and retest scapula motion.

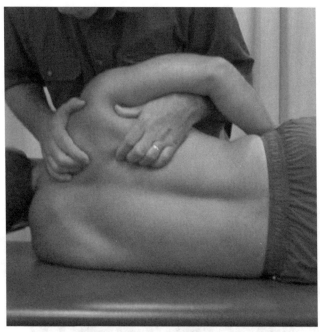

Scapula myofascial release

294

GLENOHUMERAL ABDUCTION TESTING

1. With the patient seated, grasp one or both arms at the elbow and induce passive abduction;
2. Restricted abduction can be due to restriction at the glenohumeral or acromioclavicular joint, tension in the scapula, latissimus dorsi or pectoralis muscles, and shoulder pain causing muscle guarding with movement.

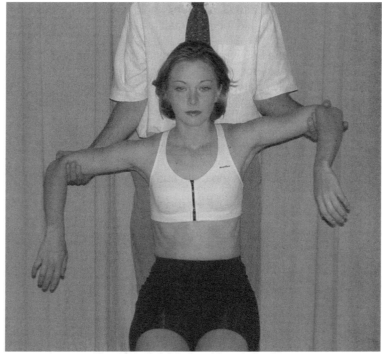

Restricted right shoulder abduction

GLENOHUMERAL MYOFASCIAL RELEASE

Indication: Glenohumeral joint restriction related to shoulder pain, arm pain, and other problems.

Relative contraindications: Acute shoulder sprain or fracture, glenohumeral joint inflammation.

Technique (supine):

1. Sit at the head of the table and firmly hold the acromioclavicular joint with one hand and the proximal forearm with your other hand;
2. Slowly abduct the arm while maintaining internal rotation, holding steady force at any restriction until tissue give is completed;
3. Slowly externally rotate the arm and move it into additional abduction, maintaining steady force at any restriction until tissue give is completed;
4. Slowly adduct the arm while maintaining external rotation, holding steady force at any restriction until tissue give is completed;
5. Slowly return the arm to the table and retest glenohumeral motion.

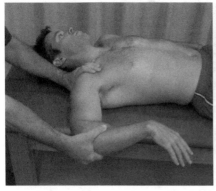 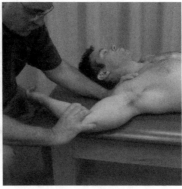

Abduction   External rotation

SPENCER TECHNIQUE (shoulder muscle energy)

Indications: Restricted shoulder motion related to shoulder pain, arm pain, back pain, chest wall pain, and other problems.

Relative contraindications: Acute fracture or dislocation, acute sprain, glenohumeral joint inflammation.

Technique (lying on opposite side):

1. Stand in front of the patient and use your cephalad hand to stabilize the acromioclavicular joint;
2. Use your other hand to test the following shoulder motions (normal range of passive motion):
   a) Extension (50°) – move the elbow posteriorly and slightly laterally;
   b) Flexion (180°) – move the elbow anteriorly and slightly medially;
   c) Circumduction with compression (smooth) – Lift the elbow to about 90° abduction, compress the elbow toward the shoulder joint, and move the elbow in small clockwise and counterclockwise circles;
   d) Circumduction with traction (smooth) – Lift the elbow or pull the wrist away from the shoulder joint and induce small clockwise and counterclockwise circles;
   e) Abduction (90° when internally rotated, 180° when externally rotated) – Place the patient's hand on your cephalad forearm and lift the elbow laterally;
   f) Internal rotation (90°) – place the back of the patient's hand behind his or her hip and pull the elbow anteriorly;
   g) Pump (smooth) – interlock your fingertips over the deltoid muscle, place the patient's hand on your shoulder, and slowly pull the arm away from the shoulder and release, repeating 5-10 times if needed;
   h) Optional additional stage: Adduction (50°) with external rotation (90°) – Place the patient's hand on your cephalad forearm and move the elbow medially across the chest;
3. If a restriction is encountered slowly move the shoulder into the barrier and ask the patient to gently push away from the restriction against your equal resistance for 3-5 seconds;
4. Slowly move the shoulder to a new restrictive barrier;
5. Repeat 3-5 times or until motion returns;
6. Retest shoulder motion.

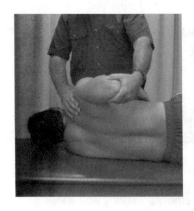

1) Extension

2) Flexion

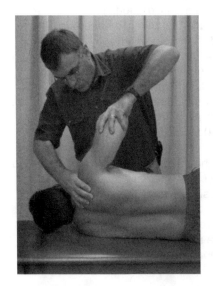

3) Circumduction/compression

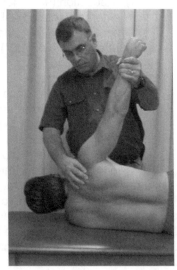

4) Circumduction/traction

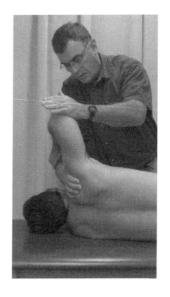

5) Abduction

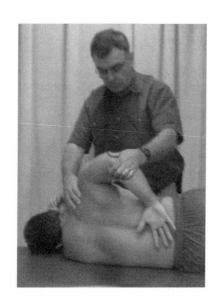

6) Internal rotation

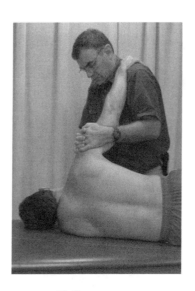

7) Pump

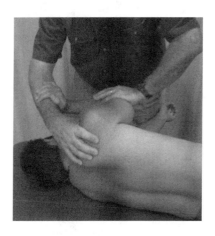

Adduction/external rotation

GLENOHUMERAL ARTICULATORY

Indication: Glenohumeral joint restriction related to shoulder pain and other problems.

Relative contraindications: Acute shoulder sprain or fracture, glenohumeral joint hypermobility or inflammation.

Technique (seated):

1. Stand behind the patient and firmly hold the acromioclavicular joint with one hand;
2. Grasp the wrist with your other hand and move the shoulder into an internal rotation and adduction barrier behind the patient's back;
3. Maintain the internal rotation barrier and slowly abduct the arm;
4. Maintain the abduction barrier and slowly externally rotate at the shoulder;
5. Slowly move the shoulder into flexion, adduction, and internal rotation barriers in an overhand throwing motion;
6. Repeat as one smooth motion 3-5 times or until joint mobility returns;
7. Retest glenohumeral motion.

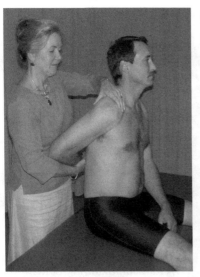 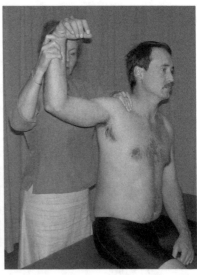

Adduction and internal rotation   Abduction and external rotation

STERNOCLAVICULAR MOTION TESTING

1. With the patient seated or supine, palpate the sternoclavicular joint and ask the patient to shrug the shoulders
   a) Superiorly to induce inferior clavicle glide;
   b) Inferiorly to induce superior clavicle glide;
   c) Anteriorly to induce posterior clavicle glide;
   d) Posteriorly to induce anterior clavicle glide;

2. Identify restrictions by comparing clavicle glide on both sides:
   Restricted inferior glide = superior clavicle;
   Restricted superior glide = inferior clavicle;
   Restricted posterior glide = anterior clavicle;
   Restricted anterior glide = posterior clavicle.

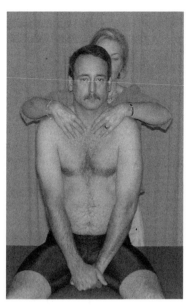

Testing inferior glide

STERNOCLAVICULAR MUSCLE ENERGY

Indications: Sternoclavicular joint restriction related to shoulder pain, chest wall pain, neck pain, and other problems.

Relative contraindications: Acute clavicle fracture, sternoclavicular joint inflammation.

Technique (supine):

1. Push or pull the medial clavicle into its restrictive barrier (exception – for superior glide restriction stabilize the opposite sternoclavicular joint);
2. Ask the patient to gently contract a muscle against your equal resistance for 3-5 seconds:
    a) Anterior clavicle – patient's flexed arm pulls posteriorly into your shoulder;
    b) Superior clavicle – patient's internally rotated arm pushes anteriorly;
    c) Inferior clavicle – patient's head rotated toward the restricted SC joint pushes into rotation away from the restricted joint;
3. Repeat 3-5 times or until motion returns;
4. Retest sternoclavicular motion.

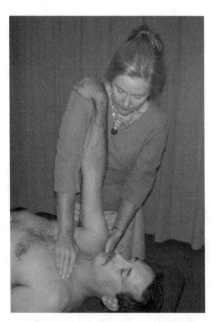

MET for right anterior clavicle

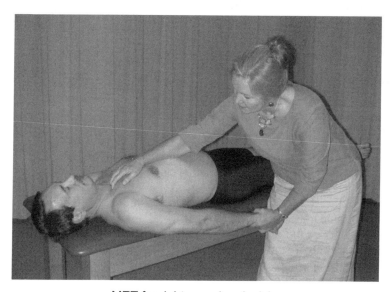

MET for right superior clavicle

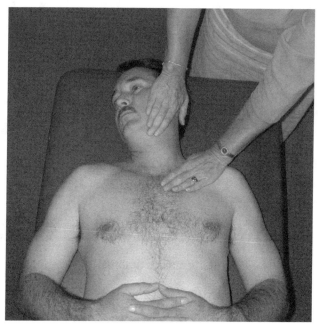

MET for right inferior clavicle

STERNOCLAVICULAR THRUST

Indications: Clavicle restricted posterior or inferior glide related to shoulder pain, chest wall pain, neck pain, and other problems.

Relative contraindications: Acute clavicle fracture or dislocation, acute shoulder sprain, sternoclavicular joint inflammation.

Technique (supine):

1. Stand on the opposite side and place the thenar eminence of your cephalad hand on the medial clavicle, pushing it in the direction of glide restriction;
2. Gap the sternoclavicular joint by placing your caudad hand on the table between the involved arm and ribs and having the patient use the other hand to pull the wrist around your forearm toward the opposite shoulder,
3. Apply a short and quick thrust into the glide restriction with your thenar eminence;
4. Retest sternoclavicular motion.

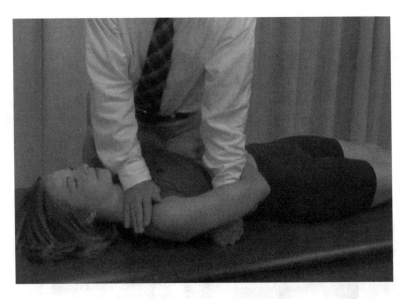

Sternoclavicular thrust

ELBOW/FOREARM EXAMINATION

1. Palpate for tenderness at the olecranon process, medial epicondyle, lateral epicondyle, and radial head. Radial head tender points are located at the anterolateral or posterolateral aspect of the radial head;
2. Palpate for tension and tenderness of the wrist flexors distal to the medial epicondyle, wrist extensors distal to the lateral epicondyle, and interosseous membrane between ulna and radius;
3. Test elbow flexion and extension to determine directions of laxity and restriction;
4. Test forearm pronation/radial head posterior glide and supination/radial head anterior glide to determine directions of laxity and restriction:
   Restricted anterior glide with supination = posterior radial head;
   Restricted posterior glide with pronation = anterior radial head.

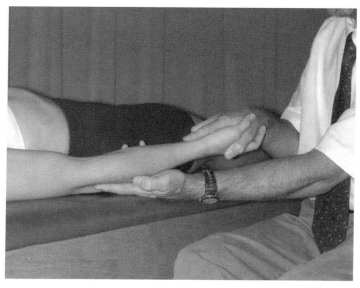

Radial head anterior glide with supination

ELBOW MYOFASCIAL RELEASE

Indication: Ulna restriction related to arm pain and other problems.

Relative contraindications: Elbow joint inflammation (direct MFR only).

Technique (seated or supine):

1. Hold the patient's hand with one hand and the proximal radius and ulna with your other hand;
2. Test elbow flexion-extension and forearm supination-pronation to determine directions of laxity and restriction;
3. Indirect: Gently and slowly move the elbow to its position of laxity, apply compression or traction between your hands to facilitate laxity, and follow any tissue release until it is completed;
4. Direct: Slowly move the elbow into its restriction and apply steady force until tissue give is completed;
5. Slowly return the elbow to neutral and retest motion.

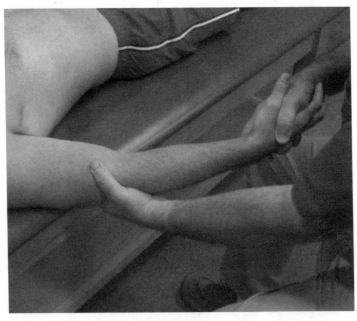

Elbow myofascial release

ELBOW PERCUSSION VIBRATOR

Indications: Ulna, radial head, or forearm somatic dysfunction associated with arm pain, elbow or forearm restriction, and other problems.

Relative contraindications: Acute elbow sprain, elbow joint inflammation, upper extremity cancer, recent elbow surgery.

Technique (supine):

1. Place your monitoring hand over the medial epicondyle;
2. Place the vibrating percussion pad lightly on the lateral epicondyle or the radial head avoiding pad bouncing;
3. Alter pad speed, pressure, and angle until vibrations are palpated as strong by the monitoring hand;
4. Maintain contact until the force and rhythm of vibration returns to that of normal tissue;
5. Alternative technique:
   a) Allow the monitoring hand to be pulled toward the pad, resisting any other direction of hand pull;
   b) Maintain percussion until the monitoring hand is pushed away from the pad;
6. Slowly release the monitoring hand and percussion vibrator and retest motion.

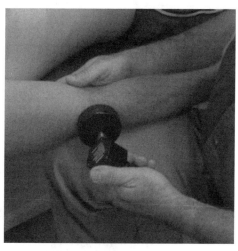

Elbow percussion vibrator

ULNA ARTICULATORY

Indication: Ulna restriction related to arm pain and other problems.

Relative contraindications: Elbow inflammation, acute elbow sprain, acute fracture, elbow joint hypermobility.

Technique (seated or supine):

1. Hold the proximal forearm with both hands, pinning the patient's hand between your arm and ribs;
2. Flex the elbow and move the ulna to a lateral glide barrier as you slowly extend the elbow;
3. Flex the elbow again and move the ulna to a medial glide barrier as you slowly extend the elbow;
4. Repeat 3-5 times or until joint mobility returns;
5. Retest elbow extension.

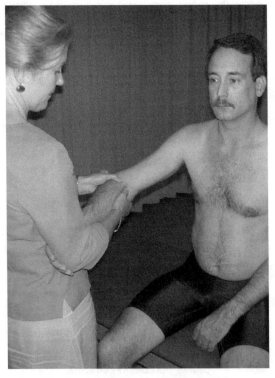

Elbow articulatory into lateral glide

RADIAL HEAD COUNTERSTRAIN

Indication: Radial head tender point associated with arm pain, forearm restriction, and other problems.

Relative contraindications: Acute radius fracture.

Technique (seated or supine):

1. Locate the tender point at the anterolateral or posterolateral head of the radius, labeling it 10/10;
2. Extend the elbow, supinate the forearm fully, and retest for tenderness;
3. Fine tune this position with slight ulna abduction or adduction until tenderness is 2/10 or less;
4. Hold the position of relief for 90 seconds;
5. Slowly and passively return the arm to neutral and retest for tenderness.

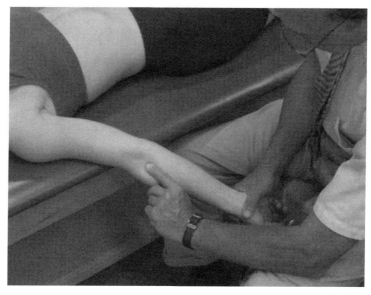

Anterior radial head tender point and treatment position

RADIAL HEAD THRUST

Indication: Restricted anterior glide of radial head associated with arm pain, forearm restriction, and other problems.

Relative contraindications: Acute sprain, acute fracture, joint inflammation.

Technique (standing, seated, or supine):

1. Hold the patient's hand and place the thumb or thenar eminence of your other hand on the posterior aspect of the radial head;
2. Gently flex the elbow and partially pronate the hand;
3. Simultaneously extend the elbow, supinate the hand, and push the radial head anteriorly to the restrictive barriers;
4. Add a short quick anterior thrust into the radial head;
5. Retest radial head motion.

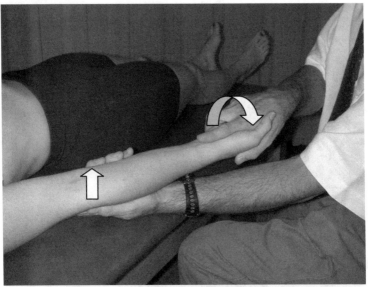

Radial head thrust

INTEROSSEOUS MEMBRANE SOFT TISSUE RELEASE

Indication: Interosseous membrane tension related to arm pain, forearm restriction, and other problems. The technique can be adapted for leg interosseous membrane tension related to leg pain, ankle restriction, and other problems.

Relative contraindications: Acute sprain, acute fracture, deep venous thrombosis.

Technique (seated or supine):

1. Palpate for tension along the ventral interosseous membrane between radius and ulna;
2. Place your thumbs over the tense area and fingers on the dorsal forearm;
3. Compress your thumbs firmly toward your fingers, adding compression or traction between your hands until tissue relaxation is completed;
4. Retest interosseous tension.

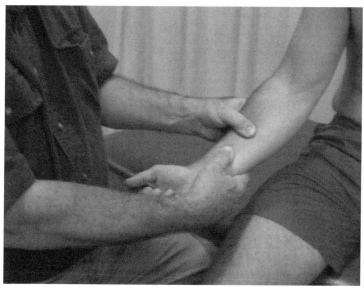

Interosseous membrane soft tissue release

311

FOREARM MUSCLE ENERGY

Indication: Restricted forearm supination or pronation associated with arm pain and other problems.

Relative contraindications: Acute sprain, acute fracture.

Technique (seated or supine):

1. Stabilize the affected elbow with one hand;
2. Hold the affected hand with your other hand and move the forearm to the restrictive barrier;
3. Ask the patient to gently turn the forearm away from the restriction against your equal resistance for 3-5 seconds;
4. Slowly move the forearm to a new restrictive barrier;
5. Repeat 3-5 times or until full motion returns;
6. Retest forearm supination and pronation.

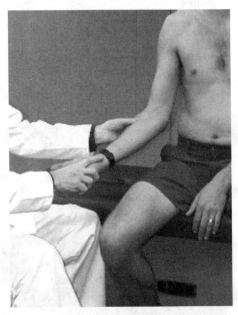

Muscle energy for restricted supination

Indication: Wrist restriction related to arm pain and other problems.

Relative contraindications: Acute sprain.

Technique (seated or supine):

1. Hold the patient's forearm with one hand and his or her hand with your other hand;
2. Test wrist abduction-adduction and flexion-extension, comparing to the other hand if needed to identify directions of laxity and restriction;
3. Indirect: Gently and slowly move the wrist to its position of laxity, apply compression or traction between your hands to facilitate laxity, and follow any tissue release until it is completed;
4. Direct: Slowly move the wrist into its restrictions and apply steady force until tissue give is completed;
5. Slowly return the wrist to neutral and retest motion.

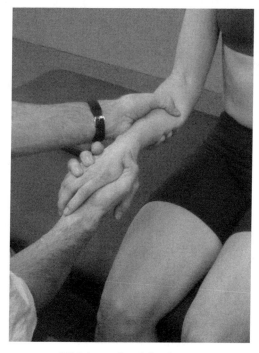

Wrist myofascial release

CARPAL TUNNEL MYOFASCIAL RELEASE

Indication: Carpal tunnel syndrome.

Relative contraindications: Acute wrist sprain, wrist inflammation.

Technique (seated or supine):

1. Hold the thumb with one hand and medial wrist with your other hand, placing your thumbs on the pisiform bone and hook of the hamate;
2. Slowly externally rotate and abduct the patient's thumb, extend the wrist, and apply steady traction between your thumbs for 5 seconds;
3. Slowly release and repeat 5-15 times.

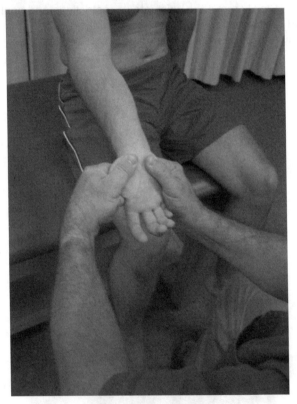

Carpal tunnel release

WRIST ARTICULATORY

Indication: Wrist restriction related to arm pain, hand pain, and other problems.

Relative contraindications: Acute sprain, wrist joint hypermobility or inflammation.

Technique (seated or supine):

1. Grasp the sides of the patient's hand with both your hands and test flexion-extension and abduction-adduction to identify restrictions;
2. Apply traction to the wrist by leaning slowly backward until the arm is straight and the wrist joint is gapped;
3. Slowly move the wrist into its position of laxity and then into its restriction while maintaining traction;
4. Repeat 3-5 times or until joint motion returns;
5. Retest wrist motion.

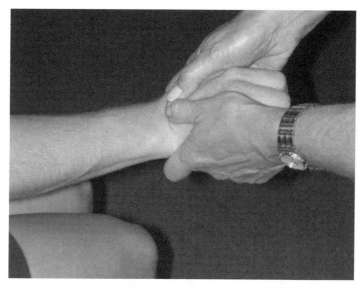

Wrist articulatory

CARPAL ARTICULATORY

Indication: Wrist restriction associated with wrist pain, hand pain, and other problems.

Relative contraindications: Acute fracture or sprain, intercarpal joint inflammation.

Technique (seated, supine, standing):

1. Grasp the wrist with both hands with your fingers interlocked and thenar or hypothenar eminences on either side of the restricted carpal bones;
2. Ask the patient to squeeze your hand, use your thenar or hypothenar eminences to compress the carpal bones, and have the patient stop squeezing;
3. Slowly circumduct the wrist clockwise and counterclockwise 3-5 times or until motion returns;
4. Repeat for other restricted carpal bones;
5. Retest wrist motion.

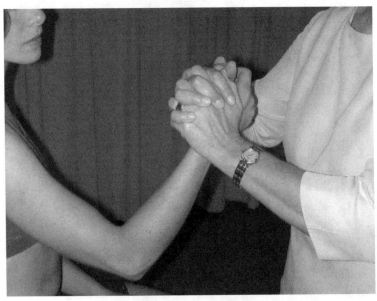

Carpal articulatory

Indication: Upper extremity somatic dysfunction associated with arm pain, restricted movement, or other problems.

Relative contraindications: Acute fracture, significant patient guarding.

Technique (supine):

1. Hold the involved arm at the hand and elbow;
2. Separate your hands to apply linear or spiral stretch to the fascia to engage a barrier;
3. Initiate horizontal or vertical oscillatory motion to the arm, feeling for restricted mobility;
4. Continue arm oscillation or modify its traction and force until you feel mobility improve.

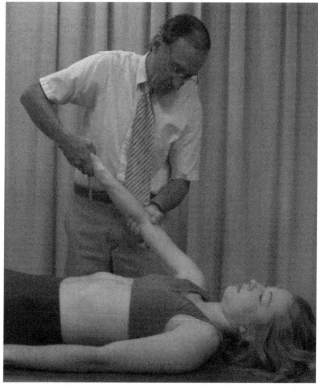

Upper extremity facilitated oscillatory release

THUMB METACARPAL THRUST

Indication: Restricted first metacarpal abduction associated with wrist pain, hand pain, and other problems.

Relative contraindications: Acute sprain, carpal-metacarpal joint hypermobility or inflammation.

Technique (seated or supine):

1. Grasp the thumb with the tip of your thumb just distal to the first carpal-metacarpal joint;
2. Use your other hand to stabilize the patient's hand;
3. Pull the metacarpal bone distally to apply traction and abduct the thumb to its restrictive barrier;
4. Apply a short and quick abduction thrust while levering the proximal metacarpal medially with your thumb;
5. Retest first metacarpal abduction.

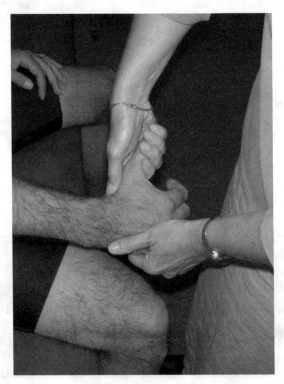

First metacarpal thrust

INTERPHALANGEAL ARTICULATORY

Indication: Interphalangeal restriction associated with hand pain and other related problems.

Relative contraindications: Acute fracture or sprain, interphalangeal joint hypermobility or inflammation.

Technique (seated or supine):

1. Stabilize the proximal bone of the joint being treated with one hand;
2. Grasp the distal bone with your other hand and gently flex and extend it to identify motion restriction;
3. Apply traction to the distal bone and slowly circumduct it in both directions 3-5 times or until motion returns;
4. Retest interphalangeal motion.

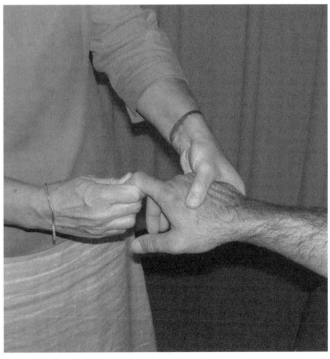

Articulatory for 2nd proximal interphalangeal joint

SHOULDER ABDUCTOR POSITION OF EASE

1. Sit with the involved arm resting on a table or counter;
2. Place one or two pillows under your arm;
3. If comfortable, take a few deep breaths and rest in this position for 2-5 minutes;
4. Repeat 2-4 times a day or as needed for pain relief.

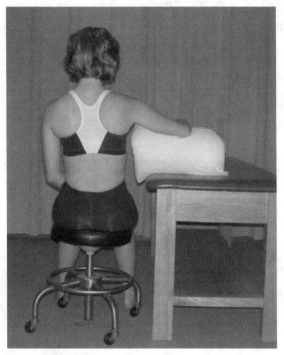

Shoulder abductor position of ease

SHOULDER ABDUCTOR STRETCH

1. Grasp the involved arm just above the elbow with the other hand;
2. Allow the involved arm to relax and use the other hand to pull it across the chest as far as it will comfortably go;
3. Take a few deep breaths and stretch for 10-20 seconds;
4. Repeat for the other arm;
5. Do this stretch 2-4 times a day.

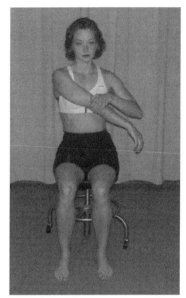

Shoulder abductor stretch

SHOULDER MOBILIZATION

1. Sit or stand with a 12-16 ounce can in the hand of the involved arm and the other arm leaning against a table or wall;
2. Allow the arm to hang freely and move the hand in small circles for 1-2 minutes;
3. Move the hand in small circles in the opposite direction for 1-2 minutes;
4. Do this mobilization 2-4 times a day.

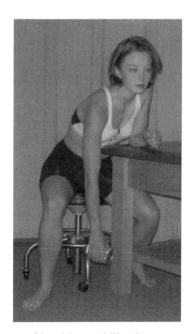

Shoulder mobilization

WRIST EXTENSOR POSITION OF EASE

1. Sit with the involved arm resting on a table or counter and your palm facing upward;
2. Place a small pillow or rolled up towel under the wrist and allow your hand to fall back over it;
3. If comfortable, take a few deep breaths and rest in this position for 2-5 minutes;
4. Repeat 2-4 times a day or as needed for pain relief.

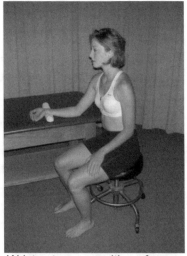

Wrist extensor position of ease

WRIST EXTENSOR STRETCH

1. Sit with the involved elbow resting on a pillow, arm straight, and hand hanging off the table with the palm facing downward;
2. Use your other hand to slowly bend the wrist downward as far as it will comfortably go;
3. Take a few deep breaths and stretch for 10-20 seconds;
4. Do this stretch 2-4 times a day.

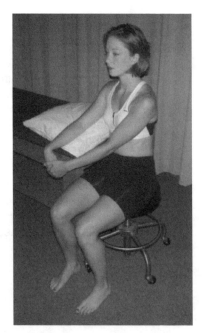

Wrist extensor stretch

RADIAL HEAD MOBILIZATION

1. Stand with the involved elbow flexed and your fist facing the upper chest;
2. Rapidly extend the elbow as far as it will go by throwing the hand forward as you simultaneously turn the fist to face upward;
3. Repeat 2-3 times if needed;
4. Do up to twice a day.

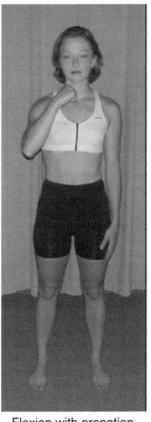
Flexion with pronation

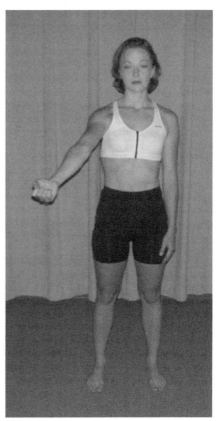
Extension with supination

CARPAL TUNNEL STRETCH[1]

1. Place your palm against a wall with the fingers pointing downward;
2. With your other hand, gently pull the thumb away from the wall;
3. Gently lean into the wall to extend the wrist as far as possible;
4. If comfortable, take a few deep breaths and stretch for 10-20 seconds;
5. Repeat for the other hand;
6. Do this stretch 2-4 times a day.

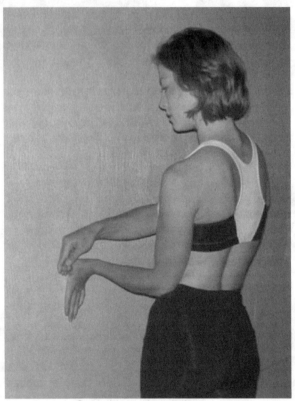

Carpal tunnel stretch

REFERENCE

1. Adapted from Sucher BM. *Palpatory diagnosis and manipulative management of carpal tunnel syndrome.* Journal of the American Osteopathic Association 94(8):647-663. 1994.

Chapter 12: VISCERAL DIAGNOSIS AND TREATMENT

Diagnosis of Visceral Somatic Dysfunction

1.   Screening – pp.330-336
   - a.   Viscerosomatic reflexes – pp.330-332
   - b.   Chapman point palpation – pp.333-336
2.   Motion testing – integrated into OMT
3.   Visceral and systemic exam as indicated
4.   Structural exam as indicated

Treatment of Visceral Somatic Dysfunction

1. OMT

Chapman point stimulation – p.333
Rib raising – pp.337-338
Thoracolumbar inhibition – p.339
Suboccipital inhibition – see p.226
Sacral rocking – see p.108
Abdominal plexus release – p.340
Abdominal sphincter release – p.341
Large intestine lift – pp.341-343
Small intestine lift – p.344
Cervicothoracic myofascial release – see pp.164-165
Thoracolumbar myofascial release – see p.163
Thoracic pump – p.345
Pectoral traction – p.346
Pedal pump – p.347
Liver/spleen pump – p.348
Upper extremity pétrissage – p.349

2. Exercises

Cervicothoracic fascia stretch – see p.247
Thoracolumbar fascia stretch – see p.147
Diaphragmatic breathing – p.350
Pectoral traction – see p.211
Pedal pump – p.350
Piston breath – p.351

VISCEROSOMATIC REFLEXES

EXAM	Acute Findings	Chronic Findings
Temperature	Hot	Cool
Tissue texture	Moisture, fullness, edema, tension	Thickness, dryness, ropiness, pimples
Red reflex	Increased or prolonged redness	Prolonged blanching

THORACOLUMBAR TEMPERATURE

1. With the patient seated or prone, hold your hand 1-2" posterior to the upper thoracic spine and slowly move it inferiorly along the spine to the upper lumbar area, noting variations in temperature;
2. Increased heat = possible acute somatic dysfunction;
3. Decreased heat or coolness = possible chronic somatic dysfunction.

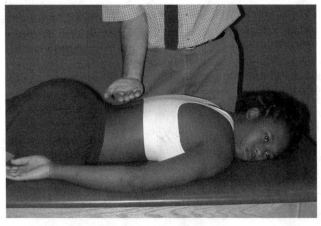

Thoracolumbar temperature

330

THORACOLUMBAR TISSUE TEXTURE

1. With the patient seated or prone, use your fingertips to palpate the thoracic and lumbar paraspinal areas from T1-L3, comparing right and left sides for skin thickness, moisture, skin drag, tension, ropiness, edema, pimples, and tenderness;
2. Moisture, fullness, edema, tension, focal tenderness = acute somatic dysfunction;
3. Thick skin, dryness, ropiness, pimples, ache = chronic somatic dysfunction.

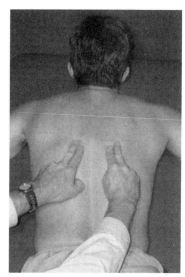

Mid-thoracic tension palpation

THORACOLUMBAR RED REFLEX

1. With the patient seated or prone, place your index and middle fingers along either side of the T1 spinous process;
2. Pressing anteriorly with just enough pressure to blanch the skin, drag your fingers along the spine to the lower lumbar area;
3. Allow a few seconds for flushing to develop and note variations in the redness pattern and in the length of time different areas remain red;
4. Increased or prolonged redness = acute somatic dysfunction;
5. Prolonged blanching = chronic somatic dysfunction.

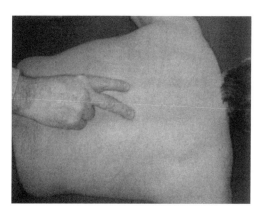

Acute upper thoracic somatic dysfunction

VISCERAL AUTONOMIC INNERVATION*

Organs	Sympathetic	Parasympathetic
Head and neck	T1-T4	Vagus
Cardiovascular	T1-T5	Vagus
Respiratory	T2-T7	Vagus
Stomach, liver, gall bladder	T5-T9	Vagus
Small intestines	T9-T11	Vagus
Ovaries, testicles	T9-T10	S2-S4
Kidney, ureters, bladder	T10-T11	S2-S4
Large intestines, rectum	T8-L2	Vagus – ascending colon S2-S4 – rest of colon
Uterus	T10-T-11	S2-S4
Prostate	L1-L2	S2-S4

* From Willard FH. Pp. 90-119 in Ward RC. *Foundations for Osteopathic Medicine, 2nd Edition.* Lippincott Williams & Wilkins, Philadelphia, 2003.

CHAPMAN POINT PALPATION

Indication: Chest wall pain, abdominal pain, thigh pain or visceral dysfunction.

1. Palpate for anterior Chapman points which are small tender nodules at the locations listed in the table and figures on subsequent pages;
2. Correlate the Chapman point with structural and visceral exam results;
3. If indicated, treat the associated posterior Chapman point with rotatory pressure for 1-30 seconds.

CHAPMAN POINT STIMULATION

Indication: Chapman point tenderness related to visceral dysfunction.

Relative contraindications: Bowel obstruction for intestinal points.

Technique (seated, prone, supine, lateral):

1. Identify a tender Chapman point by anterior or posterior palpation;
2. Use your index finger or thumb to apply rotatory pressure into the tender point for 10-30 seconds;
3. Retest for tenderness.

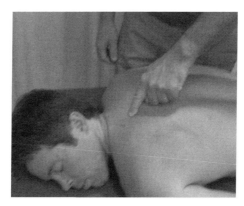

Stimulation of lower lung Chapman point

CHAPMAN POINT LOCATIONS*

Organ	Anterior Point	Posterior Point
Middle ear	Superior to medial clavicles	C1 posterior rami
Sinuses	Inferior to medial clavicles	C2 articular pillars
Pharynx	Inferior to sternoclavicular joints	C2 articular pillars
Tonsils	Medial 1st intercostal spaces	C2 articular pillars
Tongue	Medial 2nd ribs	C2 articular pillars
Esophagus, thyroid, heart	Medial 2nd intercostal spaces	T2 transverse processes
Upper lung, arm	Medial 3rd intercostal spaces	T3 transverse processes
Lower lung	Medial 4th intercostal spaces	T4 transverse processes
Liver	Right medial 5th and 6th intercostal spaces	Right T5 and T6 transverse processes
Stomach acidity	Left medial 5th intercostal space	Left T5 transverse process
Gall bladder	Right medial 6th intercostal space	Right T6 transverse process
Pancreas	Right medial 7th intercostal space	Right T7 transverse process
Spleen	Left medial 7th intercostal space	Left T7 transverse process
Small intestine	Medial 8th-10th intercostal spaces	T8-10 transverse processes
Pyloris	Midline body of sternum	T9 transverse processes
Adrenals	1" lateral and 2" superior to umbilicus	T11 transverse processes
Kidneys	1" lateral and 1" superior to umbilicus	L1 transverse processes
Bladder	Periumbilical	L2 transverse processes
Intestine peristalsis	1-2" inferior and lateral to ASIS	Between T10 and T11 transverse processes
Appendix	Tip of rib 12	Right T11 transverse process
Ovaries	Pubic tubercles	T10 transverse processes
Urethra	Pubic tubercles	L3 transverse processes
Uterus	Inferior pubic rami	L5 transverse processes
Rectum	Lesser trochanters	Lateral aspect of middle sacrum
Colon	Anterior iliotibial bands	L2-L4 transverse processes
Prostate, broad ligament	Lateral iliotibial bands	PSIS

* From Patriquin DA. Pp.1051-55 in Ward RC. *Foundations for Osteopathic Medicine, 2nd Edition.* Lippincott Williams & Wilkins, Philadelphia, 2003.

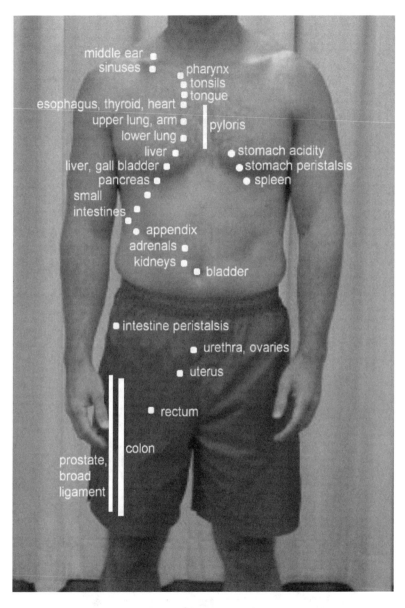

middle ear
sinuses
pharynx
tonsils
tongue
esophagus, thyroid, heart
pyloris
upper lung, arm
lower lung
liver
stomach acidity
liver, gall bladder
stomach peristalsis
pancreas
spleen
small intestines
appendix
adrenals
kidneys
bladder

intestine peristalsis
urethra, ovaries
uterus
rectum
colon
prostate, broad ligament

Anterior Chapman points
(points are bilateral unless specified in preceding table)

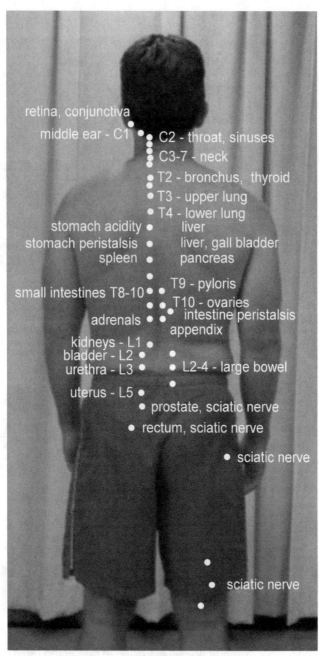

retina, conjunctiva
middle ear - C1
C2 - throat, sinuses
C3-7 - neck
T2 - bronchus, thyroid
T3 - upper lung
T4 - lower lung
stomach acidity · liver
stomach peristalsis · liver, gall bladder
spleen · pancreas
T9 - pyloris
small intestines T8-10
T10 - ovaries
intestine peristalsis
adrenals
appendix
kidneys - L1
bladder - L2
urethra - L3 · L2-4 - large bowel
uterus - L5
prostate, sciatic nerve
rectum, sciatic nerve
sciatic nerve
sciatic nerve

Posterior Chapman points

(points are bilateral unless specified in preceding table)

Indications: Rib restriction or organ dysfunction associated with sympathetic hypertonia.

Relative contraindications: Acute rib fracture, unstable cardiac arrhythmia, bowel obstruction.

Technique (supine, seated):

1. Contact the rib angles with the fingertips of both hands:
   Supine from side – reach under the arm to contact rib angles on one side;
   Supine from head – reach under the shoulders to contact rib angles on both sides;
   Seated – patient's crossed arms are draped across your shoulders, reach under arms to contact rib angles on both sides;
2. Gently push or pull the rib angles anteriorly for about 20 seconds or repetitively until rib mobility improves:
   Supine – lean your elbows into the table to facilitate rib lift;
   Seated – lean your body backward to facilitate rib lift;
3. Repeat for all of ribs 2-12 if needed.

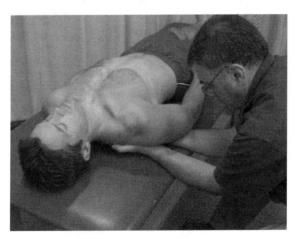

Rib raising from side

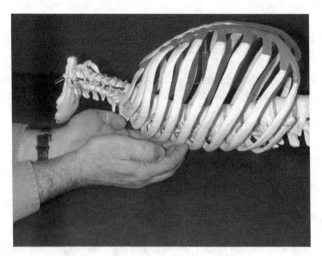

Rib raising from head (hand placement)

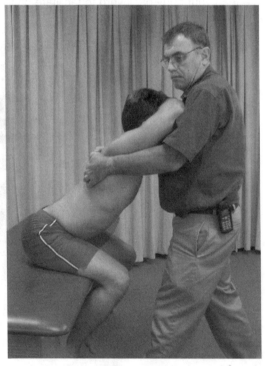

Rib raising seated

Indications: Thoracolumbar paraspinal tension associated with abdominal or pelvic disorders.

Relative contraindications: Bowel obstruction, ectopic pregnancy.

Technique (supine):

1. Sit on the side of tension and align your fingers under the tense paraspinal muscles with fingertips just lateral to the spinous processes;
2. Gently pull the muscles in an anterior and lateral direction by pushing your elbows inferiorly;
3. Maintain anterior and lateral pull on the muscles until tension is reduced;
4. Repeat for the other side if needed.

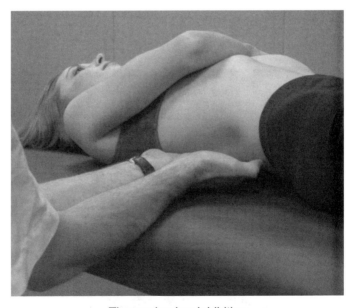

Thoracolumbar inhibition

ABDOMINAL PLEXUS RELEASE

Indications: Constipation, diarrhea, gastroesophageal reflux, cholestasis, and other functional motility problems.

Relative contraindications: Peritonitis, acute pancreatitis, abdominal aortic aneurysm, bowel obstruction, recent abdominal surgery, late pregnancy.

Technique (supine):

1. Align your fingertips from just below the xiphoid process to the umbilicus;
2. Gently press into the upper (celiac plexus), middle (superior mesenteric plexus), and lower (inferior mesenteric plexus) areas to identify tension;
3. Exert steady posterior pressure into a tense area until tension releases;
4. Retest for plexus tension.

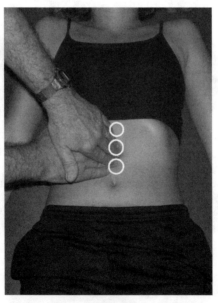

Superior mesenteric plexus release

ABDOMINAL SPHINCTER RELEASE

Indications: Constipation, gastroesophageal reflux, cholestasis, and other motility problems related to sphincter tension.

Relative contraindications: Peritonitis, appendicitis, acute cholecystitis, acute hepatitis, acute pancreatitis, splenomegaly, abdominal aortic aneurysm, bowel obstruction, recent abdominal surgery, late pregnancy.

Technique (supine):

1. Use your fingertips to gently push posteriorly and then clockwise and counterclockwise over the following sphincters to identify direction of rotational ease and restriction:
    a) Pyloric sphincter: Epigastric area 4-5 finger widths above umbilicus and slightly right of midline;
    b) Hepatopancreatic duct: Center of right upper quadrant 2-3 finger widths above umbilicus and right of midline;
    c) Duodenojejunal flexure: Center of left upper quadrant 2-3 finger widths above umbilicus and left of midline;
    d) Ileocecal valve: Center of right lower quadrant.
2. Treat the dysfunctional sphincter which has rotation opposite other sphincters with indirect or direct myofascial release:
    a) Indirect: Rotate the fascia to its position of laxity and follow any tissue release until completed;
    b) Direct: Rotate the fascia into its restriction and apply steady force until tissue give is completed;
    c) Retest fascial rotation over the dysfunctional sphincter.

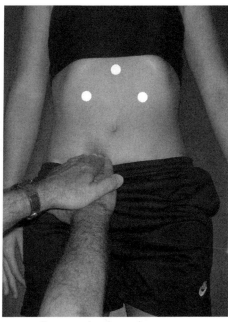

Ileocecal valve release

341

LARGE INTESTINE LIFT

Indications: Constipation, irritable bowel syndrome, and other functional disorders.

Relative contraindications: Peritonitis, colon obstruction, recent abdominal surgery.

Technique (supine):

1. Stand on the opposite side of the part of the colon being treated;
2. Reach across with the fingers of both hands and contact the lateral margin of the colon:
    Descending colon – left anterior axillary line;
    Transverse colon – above the umbilicus;
    Ascending colon – right anterior axillary line;
3. Gently lean backward to pull the colon toward its position of laxity:
    Descending and ascending colon – pull toward umbilicus;
    Transverse colon – pull toward epigastric area or umbilicus, whichever induces laxity;
4. Maintain the position of laxity and follow any tissue release until completed;
5. Gently return the colon to neutral.

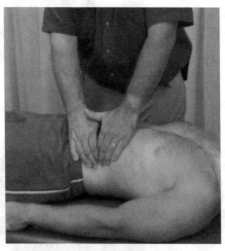

Descending colon lift

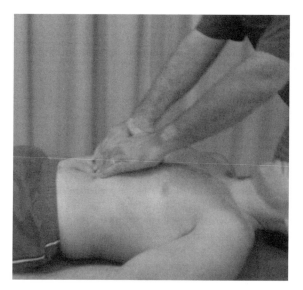

Transverse colon lift

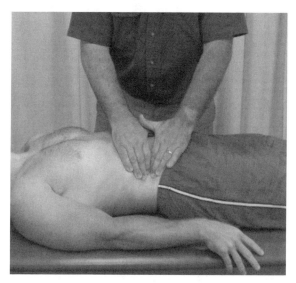

Ascending colon lift

343

SMALL INTESTINE LIFT

Indications: Indigestion, delayed gastric emptying, cholestasis, and other functional disorders.

Relative contraindications: Peritonitis, splenomegaly, recent abdominal surgery.

Technique (supine):

1. Stand to the right side of the patient, reach across with the fingers of both hands, and contact the lateral margin of the small intestine near the mid-clavicular line in the left lower quadrant;
2. Gently lean backward to pull the small intestine superomedially toward the umbilicus to its position of laxity;
3. Follow any tissue release until completed;
4. Gently return the small intestine to neutral.

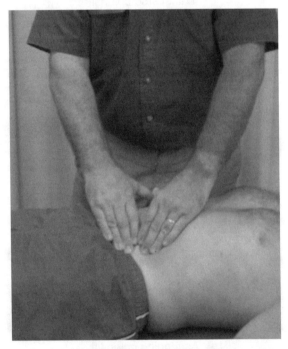

Small intestine lift

THORACIC PUMP

Indications: Atelectasis, bronchitis, pneumonia, peripheral edema, and other problems.

Relative contraindications: Acute rib fracture, severe osteoporosis, aspiration, lung cancer, pulmonary embolism, acute congestive heart failure, peritonitis, recent abdominal surgery.

Technique (supine):

1. Standing at the head of the table, place your palms on the upper chest with thumbs near the sternum and fingertips inferior to the axilla;
2. Repetitively push the upper chest posteroinferiorly at a rate and force which causes the abdomen to move up and down, about a hundred pumps per minute;
3. Continue pumping for 1/2-2 minutes as tolerated;
4. Alternative technique:
   a) Ask the patient to take deep breaths and during exhalation repetitively pump at a rate and force which causes the abdomen to move up and down;
   b) With inhalation maintain steady compressive pressure on the upper chest;
   c) Repeat the exhalation pump and inhalation resistance for several breaths as tolerated;
   d) During the early part of the last inhalation suddenly release hand pressure to encourage rapid lung expansion and increased venous and lymphatic return.

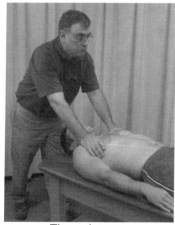
Thoracic pump

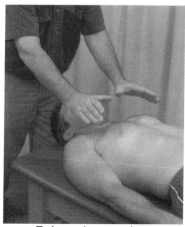
Rebound expansion

PECTORAL TRACTION

Indications: Atelectasis, bronchitis, pneumonia, peripheral edema, and other problems.

Relative contraindications: Aspiration, acute rib fracture.

Technique (supine):

1. Sit or stand at the head of the table and firmly grasp the lateral border of the pectoralis muscles at the anterior axillary folds;
2. Slowly lean backward to stretch the pectoralis muscles;
3. Ask the patient to take deep breaths and during inhalation increase pectoralis stretch, maintaining steady traction during exhalation;
4. Continue until tissue give is completed and then slowly release traction.

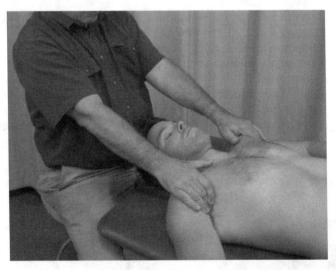

Pectoral traction

PEDAL PUMP

Indications: Peripheral edema, atelectasis, bronchitis, pneumonia, and other problems.

Relative contraindications: Acute ankle sprain, acute congestive heart failure, lymphatic cancer, deep venous thrombosis, peritonitis, recent abdominal surgery.

Technique (supine):

1. Standing at the foot of the table, place your palms on the plantar surface of the feet with fingers over the toes;
2. Dorsiflex the feet to the restrictive barrier to stretch the fascia of the posterior compartment of the leg;
3. Repetitively lean into your palms to rhythmically dorsiflex the ankles at a rate and force which causes the abdomen to move up and down, about a hundred pumps per minute;
4. Alternative technique: Hold the dorsal surface and repetitively pull the ankles into plantar flexion;
5. Continue pumping for 1/2-2 minutes as tolerated.

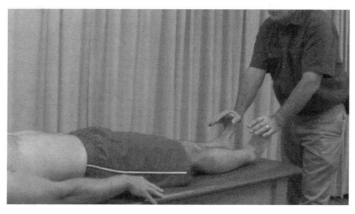

Dorsiflexion pump

LIVER/SPLEEN PUMP

Indications: Liver, gall bladder, or spleen dysfunction.

Relative contraindications: Acute hepatitis, acute cholecystitis, peritonitis, undiagnosed hepatomegaly or splenomegaly.

Technique (supine):

1. Place one hand on the costal margin overlying the involved organ and your other hand under the ribs posterior to the organ;
2. Gently compress the ribs between your hands until tissue give stops;
3. Have the patient take a deep breath and during exhalation repetitively compress the ribs between your hands using gentle force;
4. During early inhalation quickly release hand pressure to cause rib recoil;
5. Repeat the exhalation pump and inhalation recoil 3-5 times if tolerated.

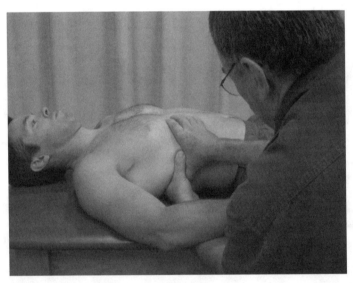

Liver pump

UPPER EXTREMITY PETRISSAGE

Indications: Upper extremity edema.

Relative contraindications: Lymphatic or metastatic cancer, deep venous thrombosis, compartment syndrome.

Technique (lateral):

1. Place the patient's hand on your shoulder and interlock your fingers on the upper arm;
2. Gently squeeze the tissues and exert counterclockwise and clockwise motion toward the shoulder, repeating 3-5 times;
3. Grasp the arm above the elbow, gently squeeze the tissues, and exert counterclockwise and clockwise motion toward the shoulder, repeating 3-5 times;
4. Grasp the forearm just below the elbow, gently squeeze the tissues, and exert counterclockwise and clockwise motion toward the elbow, repeating 3-5 times;
5. Grasp the forearm just above the wrist, gently squeeze the tissues, and exert counterclockwise and clockwise motion toward the elbow, repeating 3-5 times.

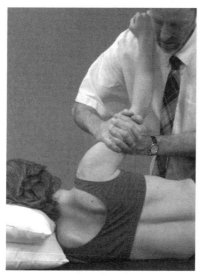
Arm pétrissage

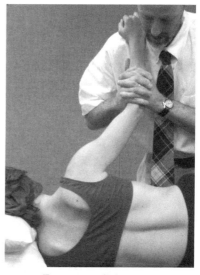
Forearm pétrissage

DIAPHRAGMATIC BREATHING

1. Lie on your back with knees bent and a hand resting on the lower abdomen;
2. Slowly take a deep breath all the way in, allowing your abdomen to rise during inhalation;
3. Slowly let your breath all the way out, allowing the abdomen to drop during exhalation;
4. Repeat 5-10 times;
5. Do this exercise 2-4 times a day or as often as needed.

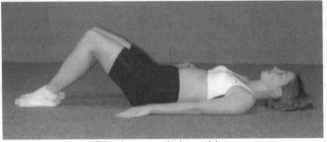

Diaphragmatic breathing

PEDAL PUMP

1. Lie on your back with knees bent and toes against a wall;
2. Rapidly push your feet into the wall and release to move your abdomen up and down;
3. Repeat about twice a second for 1/2-2 minutes;
4. Do this pump 2-4 times a day as needed.

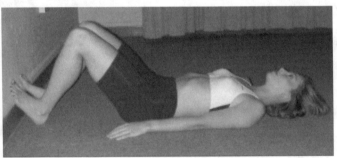

Pedal pump

350

PISTON BREATH[1]

1. Sit upright with the arms hanging at your sides;
2. Push your shoulders backward and turn your hands outward as far as they will go, creating tension in your upper chest;
3. Breath deeply in and out through the nose using brisk but steady breaths without pause between cycles;
4. With each exhalation allow the shoulders to move farther back and the arms to turn more outward;
5. Repeat for 10 breaths, pacing yourself to avoid lightheadedness;
6. Do once a day, gradually increasing the number of breaths.

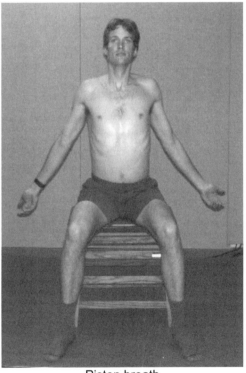

Piston breath

REFERENCE

1. Adapted from Comeaux ZC. *Robert Fulford, D.O. and the Philosopher Physician*. Eastland Press, Seattle, 2002.

Osteopathic manipulative treatment has a major role in primary care practices in which functional complaints such as back pain, headache, neck symptoms, cough, upper respiratory congestion, abdominal pain, and leg symptoms are among the most frequent reasons for patient visits.[1] Integration of OMT into a busy practice requires examination and treatment skills that are time efficient and efficacious. The following treatment models have been successful at streamlining osteopathic diagnosis and treatment for primary care.

Region of complaint is the first cue many osteopathic physicians use to determine if there is related somatic dysfunction. However, problems which persist after an initial treatment may need to be evaluated for somatic dysfunction in a region on either side of the chief complaint. Chronic problems often require more detailed exam for systemic, postural, or multi-factorial problems.

Chronic low back pain has been associated with six somatic dysfunctions termed the **dirty half dozen**[2]:

1) Non-neutral lumbar (single segment);
2) Pubic compression or shear;
3) Extended sacrum (backward torsion or unilateral extension);
4) Innominate shear (downslip, upslip, unilateral sacral flexion);
5) Short leg/sacral base unleveling;
6) Muscle imbalance of trunk or lower extremities.

Evaluation for these causes of chronic low back pain can be achieved by selected palpation and motion testing. Landmarks for palpation include ASIS, pubic symphysis, PSIS, sacral base and ILA, lumbar transverse processes, and tender points for iliacus, piriformis, and iliolumbar ligaments. Motion testing for sacroiliac joints, sacrum, and lumbar spine completes the diagnosis. Treatment of the identified cause with OMT, flexibility exercises, and postural strengthening can help some people afflicted with failed low back syndrome.

Upper back pain can be efficiently evaluated by palpatory screening for **single segment** and key rib somatic dysfunctions. Paravertebral fullness, spasm, or rotation restriction at one vertebral level is more often causative of pain than group somatic dysfunctions. Treatment of a single segment restriction (type 2, non-neutral) will often resolve surrounding group dysfunctions.

Chest wall pain is frequently associated with a **key rib** somatic dysfunction. The key rib is that which, when treated, resolves other rib tender points or motion restrictions. Rib somatic dysfunctions linked to a key rib include:

Inhalation group – Inferior rib;
Exhalation group – Superior rib;
Multiple rib tender points – Anterior or posterior subluxed rib;
Bilateral rib somatic dysfunction – Corresponding thoracic vertebra.

Treatment of a related thoracic dysfunction may resolve rib somatic dysfunction. If not, treatment of the key rib instead of all ribs can significantly reduce treatment time.

Chronic headache has been related to **cervical and non-physiological cranial somatic dysfunctions**. Persistent occipitoatlantal, atlantoaxial, and typical cervical joint restrictions can be treated to help some people with chronic tension headaches. Sphenobasilar compressions, vertical strains, or lateral strains are diagnosed by palpation of sphenoid greater wings and occiput during cranial flexion and extension. Treatment of these cranial base somatic dysfunctions can be achieved with sphenobasilar compression-decompression or balanced membranous tension techniques.

Multi-region or systemic dysfunctions can be efficiently diagnosed and treated using **fascial patterns**.[3] Four transverse fascial diaphragms can be quickly tested with the patient supine and categorized as ideal (no restriction), compensated (alternating restrictions), or uncompensated (not alternating). The fascial diaphragms and their corresponding fascial exam and vertebrae are:

1) Pelvic diaphragm – Lumbosacral fascia – L5-S1;
2) Thoracic diaphragm – Thoracolumbar fascia – T12-L3;
3) Thoracic inlet – Cervicothoracic fascia – C7-T4;
4) Foramen magnum – Occipitoatlantal fascia – OA-C2.

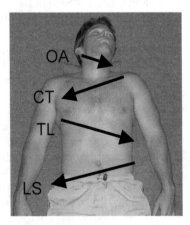

Common compensatory pattern

Treatment of the uncompensated or restricted fascial diaphragms or corresponding vertebral segments with myofascial release or thrust can improve overall postural compensation, lymphatic drainage, and recovery from illness.

The primary care application of osteopathic diagnosis and treatment is what appears to distinguish osteopathic medicine but the application of these skills is guided by an underlying philosophy. In the words of Marlene A. Wager, DO, Professor of Family Medicine at WVSOM:

> "The philosophy of treating the body as a whole, the holistic approach to patients, the knowledge that the body can heal itself, especially if in true alignment which can be accomplished by manipulation of the musculoskeletal system ... this is osteopathic medicine."

REFERENCES

1. American Academy of Family Physicians. *2005 FACTS About Family Practice.* http://www.aafp.org/x530.xml. 2005.
2. Greenman PE. *Principles of Manual Medicine, 2nd Edition.* Lipincott Williams & Wilkins, Baltimore, 1996.
3. Kuchera ML, Kappler RE. *Clinical significance of fascial patterns.* Pp.583-584 in Ward RC. *Foundations for Osteopathic Medicine, 2nd Edition.* Lippincott Williams & Wilkins, Philadelphia, 2003.

INDEX

Note: Page numbers with a *t* indicate tables.

367